# Keys to Survival

# Keys to Survival

Irene McCullough Pace

# Contents

To my husband Amos,
*the right man for the job!*

and

*To the memory of the millions of women
who died asking: "Why didn't someone tell us
about the cause of this disease?"*

And I will give unto thee the keys of the kingdom of heaven: and whatsoever thou shall bind on earth shall be bound in heaven; and whatsoever thou shall loose on earth shall be loosed in heaven.

*Matthew 16:19*

# Advance praise for *Keys to Survival*:

❧ Pace's *Keys to Survival* is a journey of courage, faith and grace. Her story should be read by all women.—Rev. Dr. Susan Newman, author of *Oh God! A Black Woman's Guide to Sex and Spirituality*

❧ *Keys to Survival* is a compelling story that gives insight into a horrific disease, a wonderful marriage, and an unfailing belief in God. A realistic look at cervical cancer from a patient's point of view, *Keys* gives an inside look at the trials and tribulations from discovery through treatment, relates the impact on family and friends, and shows that even the darkest cloud contains a silver lining. God bless you, Irene, for having the intestinal fortitude to expose your underbelly, and for letting us accompany you as you relive your journey through this major life experience.—*Robin L. Maxwell, RPh, Former Vice President, New Jersey State Pharmacists Association*

❧ By sharing her experience, Irene Pace reveals the very high toll cervical cancer exacts. *Keys to Survival* shows what diagnosis and treatment feel like and exposes the impact on family, friends, and society as a whole. Thank God for the Christian perspective. This story is long overdue for women of all ages.—*Myika Dunn, RN, MSN, former Clinical Nursing Instructor, University of Pennsylvania School of Nursing*

❧ *Keys to Survival* challenges readers of all ages to think twice about the long-term consequences of HPV infection, cervical cancer, and lifestyle choices that increase the risk of disease.—*Mark Morgan, M.D.*

# Acknowledgments

Thanks be to God who always gives us the victory through our Lord Jesus Christ.

*Keys to Survival* is a personal chronicle filled with intimate details about a sensitive topic. There is no way to experience or tell such a story without the help of countless individuals. I am especially grateful to all who allowed me to use their names in this book. Your good name means everything to me. I believe God used the silent unnamed individuals who played a crucial role during diagnosis, treatment, and beyond in ways that defy description. I applaud you. At the risk of inadvertent omissions, I acknowledge several groups of people whose love, prayers, support and encouragement are deeply appreciated.

For the past fifteen years, I've called New Jersey "home." Before that, I lived on the West Coast, in New England, in the Midwest, and in the nation's capital. I am blessed to call many hardworking professionals, business owners, and community leaders my friends and neighbors. I praise God for your love and friendship, and that of your children.

During these years in South Jersey, at various times I've called three unique places my "church home." I have also found joy in congregational worship at churches in California, Rhode Island, and Massachusetts. Each offered a different worship style. Each taught me to serve the Lord Jesus with gladness. Each brought new and exciting opportunities for fellowship. Brothers and sisters in Christ, I praise God for your prayers and compassion. Asbury United Methodist Church is very special . . . called for such a time as this.

When the news wasn't good, I needed doctors, nurses, and pharmacists. I owe a debt of gratitude to the medical specialists and their support staffs who treated me with professionalism and warmth. I also applaud the commitment of the pastoral care community. I learned so much from cancer patients and their families who welcomed me into their hospital rooms as a volunteer chaplain long before my own diagnosis. I am especially grateful to those who encouraged me to write about my experiences, and who are at the forefront of gynecological cancer education and research.

I extend special thanks to staff members at Borders Books and Xlibris. Their pilot professional publishing program enabled me to bring *Keys* to light with editorial freedom. Just what the doctor ordered!

Stonecroft, Inc. is an international, interdenominational Christian outreach group headquartered in Missouri. I'm a certified speaker for Stonecroft and serve South Jersey Women's Connection, my local organization. Thank you, SJWC. You are an energetic group of gracious, faithful women whose prayers and support mean more than mere words can say. Thank you, Stonecroft, for the training to share my testimony of Christ's power to change hearts and transform lives. Thank you, Stonecroft host families, for your love and hospitality during speaking engagements.

We choose our friends, but God chooses our family. I love you, McCullough clan. I love you, Pace people. Thanks, dear daughters, for all your love, laughter, and music. I hope I've learned to "pace" myself because marriage not only changed my last name. It changed my life. God Himself gave me the right man for the job!

# Introduction

I sat bewildered in the last row of a quiet, empty sanctuary. I was confused and full of self-pity, heavy hands cradling a weary head. *What's going to happen to me?*

Stone-cold panic and a crippling fear had ripped me apart two weeks earlier, creating a deep and debilitating depression. Powerful antidepressants numbed the mind I prized. Once a promising journalist, now I couldn't sleep but didn't want to get out of bed. I hit rock bottom back in 1980.

Looking toward the front of the church on this dismal day, I recognized the empty cross as if I was seeing it for the very first time. Sitting there, I realized Jesus Christ had suffered and died for me personally . . . for my sins, guilt, and shame. The empty cross gave me hope. That moment marked my personal belief that Jesus died for me and rose from the grave for me.

By the time the story of *Keys to Survival* began to unfold in November 2000, I enjoyed a time-tested track record of trusting Jesus, praying, and believing to see my prayers answered. I share this cancer journey:

1. to encourage readers to place their faith and trust in Jesus Christ;
2. to demonstrate that it *is* possible to experience peace, mercy, and even joy through life's trials; and
3. to jar women out of complacency and a false sense of security regarding their reproductive health.

Cervical cancer can impact women of all ages . . . from sexually active teenagers to menopausal grandmothers. By breaking the silence about this illness, I hope to inform those who might otherwise remain clueless to potential cervical troubles on the horizon.

Irene McCullough Pace
June 2004

# Part I

## The Diagnosis

# Chapter 1

## The Unexpected Symptom

**⊸ Beloved, do not think it strange concerning the fiery trial which is to try you . . .**

*1 Peter 4:12*

The pulsating spray jabbed my skin like a thousand tiny pin pricks. Immediately, I dodged the water's full force, then reached overhead to adjust the setting. Weary muscles needed more moderate stimulation today. Pounding water eased tensions from my neck, shoulders and upper back. Poised to enjoy my first Parent's Weekend at Cornell University, I showered in leisurely preparation for dinner with Professors Sandra Greene and Kodjopa Attoh. The blessing of meeting this husband and wife team could not be measured. I knew no one in Ithaca. Friendly contacts to help my daughter Lorraine if the need arose were invaluable. Although we had never met, Sandra graciously extended an invitation to spend Friday evening with her family. She and I became acquainted via email after my neighbors learned our oldest daughter planned to attend Cornell. Bob and Linda Harris set the wheels in motion. Friends since childhood, Bob and Sandra grew up in Ohio. Sandra suggested I contact the Ithaca Bed and Breakfast Association for local lodgings. I appreciated her recommendation and thanked God for someone who knew the ropes.

Now, I relished the soothing warmth, incessant pounding, and sound of the cascading waterfall. Slippery, fragrant soap slipped from my grasp and just missed my big toe. *No freak home accidents today. Too much has happened to make this day possible,* I mused. With the freedom of a playful child on a rainy summer day, I lathered and splashed with total abandon. Finally, I could unwind, relax, and salvage a few precious moments for myself.

*I'm singing in the rain,* I hummed softly. "What a mighty God we serve," I caroled.

*Dear heavenly Father, this is wonderful. You alone have put this together. I know it! Thank you so much. I love you, Lord.*

The morning traffic on the Walt Whitman Bridge into Philadelphia flowed smoothly that first Friday in November 2000. Once the car trunk slammed, there was no turning back. By timing the departure to avoid the rush hour, the towering bridge spans came into view around nine o'clock. In minutes, the car rounded the curve along the interstate and passed the stately art museum with its imposing Doric columns. The Schuylkill River sparkled, a picturesque foreground for the charming cottages along Boathouse Row. Breezing northeast on the Pennsylvania Turnpike, my husband Amos accelerated to pass a caravan of eighteen-wheelers. Could he possibly shave time off the four-hour drive from New Jersey to Ithaca? Well before we crossed the state line into upstate New York, my fifteen-year-old daughter Dana settled into her backseat groove and nodded in rhythm to music piped through CD headphones. Along the way, I gasped in awe at the breathtaking spectacle of the remaining autumn foliage. "Ithaca is Gorges," the bumper stickers and tee shirts proclaimed. Nestled in the beautiful Finger Lakes region of upstate New York, Cornell University is the gem of the Ivy League. The sprawling campus sparkles like a diamond atop black velvet . . . a precious jewel in the middle of nowhere. The day was warm, clear, and dry . . . perfect weather to embrace the promise of a truly memorable fall weekend.

I welcomed God's presence. That's *His* specialty: showing up right on time and making a way out of no way. In mid-April, Lorraine weighed college acceptances while Amos and I sharpened our pencils to calculate tuition payments. Through the process, the Lord assured me: *I call things that are not as though they were.* By His grace alone she left for Cornell in August with a generous financial aid package that included a paltry student loan to offset more than $32,000 for tuition, room, and board. In late September, God showed His hand of mercy again. After Amos and I finally made a belated commitment to attend Parent's Weekend, we discovered all local hotels booked solid. Again, God's reminder— *my grace is sufficient*—calmed my fears.

Since the local hotels anticipated a deluge of parents on pilgrimage, I called the bed-and-breakfast association for weekend accommodations as Sandra suggested. I had never arranged bed-and-breakfast lodgings before, so I must admit I was skeptical at first. The association wanted $450 for a two-bedroom, two-bath condo, payable in two installments by mid-October. With no hope of a hotel reservation within a fifty-mile radius, procrastination was costly.

"Do you think the owner would be willing to accept $425?" I asked. "Do you have the names of some references?" I inquired.

I spoke briefly with a woman who rented the condo during the summer. She assured me the lovely home fit her needs perfectly. Still somewhat reluctant but blessed with the guts to suggest a slightly lower rate, I sent the required deposit. I missed Lorraine. A few dollars wasn't going to prevent me from visiting my daughter. This was my chance to show visible support just like I did during her elementary and high school years.

Within a few days after sending the final payment, I received the homeowner's name and directions to the property. The letter instructed me to telephone a week prior to arrival and arrange to pick up the door keys. The owner and I exchanged phone pleasantries for a few minutes, and then she dropped the bombshell. I'd find the door key under the jug on the front porch when I arrived. Although I'd lived in suburban communities for nearly twenty years, I remained a city girl at heart, raised to take precautions on Chicago's crime-plagued West Side. In the 'hood, nobody in their right mind left keys anywhere near the front door.

"The jug? Is it safe?" I stammered. "Is there a neighbor you could trust with your keys?" I asked hopefully.

"Oh, that's what I always do. Everything will be perfectly fine," Sara, the owner, assured me. "And just leave the keys under the jug when you leave on Sunday," she added.

I pictured Amos' raised eyebrows and anticipated his questions. After twenty-five years of marriage, I knew this man reared in poverty-stricken Chester, Pennsylvania. What if the plan mysteriously backfired? What then, after a four-hour drive from New Jersey?

True to form, Amos balked when informed of the arrangements.

"What are we going to do if the key isn't under the jug?"

"It'll be there," I responded. Nothing could dissuade me from affirming God's presence or provision. "God's got this."

When we arrived, a turn of the key ushered us into a tastefully decorated two-story townhouse with a gorgeous upstairs view overlooking a scenic gorge. Located about fifteen minutes from Cornell's campus, the serene location just up the hill past Ithaca College could not have been more convenient. Once inside, I dropped to my knees in the living room and praised the Lord Jesus. Dana carried her suitcase and book bag to the sunny upstairs bedroom. She expressed her opinion without hesitation: "This is so much better than a cramped hotel room."

Our gracious host had left a cordial note of welcome alongside a box of delicious pastries and bagels. In addition, Sara stocked the refrigerator with everything we could ever want to eat or drink. Filled with decorative and whimsical touches throughout, the spacious townhouse afforded a very comfortable weekend retreat.

I dialed Lorraine's number after a cursory inspection of our temporary living quarters.

"Hi, Rain. We made it safely. You should see this place. It's beautiful."

Openly enthusiastic about our visit, she suggested we head over to her dormitory to meet some of her friends, and then eat lunch at a place called Wegman's.

Lunch at a grocery-store food court didn't sound too exciting, but I was game for anything Lorraine wanted. Amos maneuvered through the crowded parking lot. Inside the store, proud parents opened their wallets for tousled sons and disheveled daughters. Distinct aromas and delectable flavors intermingled in infinite array and unparalleled variety. Knowledgeable staff wearing short white jackets and bouffant chef hats directed the uninitiated who blocked traffic. Four-star service diminished any concern for the crowd. What a blessing to hear Lorraine and Dana chattering away like magpies again. Dana missed Lorraine too. Though three years apart in age, the sisters remained close friends and looked amazingly like identical twins. Some days even I couldn't tell them apart.

After lunch, Lorraine toured our weekend hideaway. We talked and laughed between mouthfuls of dessert, then Amos and Lorraine drove to her dorm with plans to return around 5:45 that evening.

Before showering, I peered down from the second-floor balcony overlooking the vaulted living room and surveyed the landscape. Dana was right: this was ten thousand times better than a hotel room. Amos had reclined in the oversized upholstered corner chair, propped his legs on the ottoman, and fallen asleep. I understood the toll of cramming five full workdays into a scant four this week. Oblivious to everything except the remote control in one hand and a gooey pastry in the other, Dana sprawled comfortably on the living room sofa. I watched unnoticed as she surfed channels to find the MTV station.

I turned away to peruse a four-shelf bookcase overflowing with framed photographs. *Sara must have a big family,* I thought. I couldn't resist the appeal of a gigantic brown teddy bear seated on the balcony's cozy full-size sofa. I hugged this furry friend with the pudgy belly. The oversized bear slumped like a sentry just off guard duty. I joined him.

Now, I flung open the pastel shower curtain with an elaborate flourish. Unhurried for the first time in weeks with almost two hours before dinner, I felt relaxed. The seashell motif and lighthouse accessories enhanced my mood. I stepped from the shower dripping with contentment. Steamy swirls of mist obscured the mirror, but not my focus. I planned to look casually elegant in an ankle-length black knit sweater dress and low-heeled black suede shoes. The late-fall weather was uncharacteristically balmy. I wouldn't even need a coat. I used the bathroom before applying lotion to damp skin. A slight tinge of blood on the tissue surprised me.

"For crying out loud," I moaned with exasperation. *Not today. Not now.* The onset of my monthly period caught me completely off guard. It wasn't due until Monday.

*Lord, have mercy. Can you believe this? We were just at the grocery store.*

Just like clockwork since I was thirteen years old, my periods normally arrived at regular twenty-six-day intervals. *What a royal pain,* I thought, as I searched under the sink. Naturally, there wasn't a tampon or sanitary pad in sight.

I wrapped a towel around my midsection and headed downstairs.

"Thank you, Lord," I whispered after finding the necessary feminine protection under the sink in the first-floor bathroom. I mouthed the words "thank you, Jesus" as I returned upstairs, but no one heard except my heavenly Father. *When we pick up Lorraine before dinner, I'll get some pads from her,* I thought as I applied makeup. It must be all the excitement of the weekend, I figured, explaining away the unexpected discharge. The nonstop pace of the past week . . . running around, putting everything in place before leaving town, had been relentless. *That's all it is . . . the stress of this week,* I thought. But that's behind me now. I fluffed the pillows and slipped between the printed sheets. What better time to reflect on God's goodness and mercy?

For starters, Lorraine had made us all very proud and extremely grateful. We cheered when she opened the letter with news of over $20,000 in scholarships including a prestigious Cornell Tradition Fellowship. I remembered late April again. Two days before mailing the required deposit to Cornell, Amos got a pink slip. The layoff notice was not totally unwelcome. His job as project engineer on Denver's high-tech toll road, E-470, placed tremendous strain on me. In eighteen months of commuting from New Jersey to Colorado the frequent flyer miles added up quickly. Frankly, I praised God and steadfastly affirmed He knew the plans for Amos and the rest of us throughout the three months he remained jobless. I rejoiced to still be counted among the cheerful givers . . . to our church fellowship, the mortgage company, the gasoline station, the grocery store, our insurance agents, and now, the $1,400 monthly installment for college tuition. As first-generation college graduates in both of our families, Amos and I realized Lorraine's achievement and this prospective weekend opened an exciting new vista for the next generation of our family.

By the time we left the Attohs', Sandra and I shared an unexpected connection. Sandra completed graduate studies at Northwestern University, my alma mater. Ironically, her undergraduate choice was Kalamazoo College in Michigan, a school I declined, although I often imagined it would have been the perfect fit for me. Sandra exuded warmth and a gracious hospitality. We laughed about the challenges of raising teenagers and passed the bowl for second helpings of African rice and spicy chicken.

The next morning, a lavish university-sponsored buffet for families of freshmen Tradition Fellows hit the spot. I thoroughly enjoyed the honor bestowed on Lorraine, and the conversation with other students, parents, and faculty at our dining table. For entertainment, one of Cornell's *a cappella* male chorus groups performed a spirited medley showcasing their repertoire and range. Next, we toured the campus before the afternoon football kick-off. I felt a little tired after the morning meal, but still cheered wildly for Big Red despite the intermittent annoying ooze of the vaginal discharge. After dinner I didn't have to twist any arms to attend the Saturday evening wind ensemble concert. Afterward, I dragged tired feet to the parked car.

Sunday morning dawned so quickly. Amos loaded the car while Dana double-checked for forgotten items upstairs. I closed the front door and tucked the key safely under the jug. We looked high and low for a parking space to attend one of the campus worship services, to no avail. I had hoped to slip discretely into a back pew, but there wasn't a parking space in sight. Shortly after breakfast, it was time to hit the road again. Lorraine seemed happy about her dorm and new friends. Life without a roommate certainly had its privileges. At curbside, I hugged that girl and thanked God for her adjustment to college life.

"See you at Thanksgiving," I called as Amos drove away.

On Monday morning, my period started right on schedule and ran its normal five-day course. The watery discharge tinged with blood returned Saturday night, however. Monday morning, I called the office of Dr. Linda Stanley, my gynecologist for the past five years. Unfortunately, she was out of town. The receptionist offered the earliest available appointment with Dr. Stanley's associate, another female gynecologist. She had an opening Thursday, one week before Thanksgiving. The young gynecologist listened intently as I recited my symptoms. She conducted a pelvic exam, but no Pap test. Dr. Stanley performed my last Pap test in January, ten months ago. The results: normal. Now, the doctor prescribed a five-day supply of metronidazole, an antibacterial vaginal gel to be used with a small applicator for the next five nights. If the discharge continued, the next step involved an endometrial biopsy, the removal of a small sampling of tissues from the lining of the uterus, she explained. When I left the office, I didn't give the biopsy even a second thought. Like many people, I associate biopsies with cancer. But I didn't have cancer. No one in my family had cancer. I would simply fill the prescription, use this messy stuff, and be done. *The sooner the better,* I thought. I was sick and tired of sanitary pads.

After I faithfully used the medication, the watery discharge tinged with blood returned the day before Thanksgiving. I called the doctor's office the following Monday to schedule an appointment for the endometrial biopsy, a relatively painless ten-minute office procedure. When I arrived on Tuesday, December 5, the receptionist seemed surprised.

"We wondered what happened to you," she said.

Her appointment book told the story. She pointed to my penciled name on Monday, December 4. I mistakenly confused the dates and showed up a day late for the evening appointment. Yet another week of the watery discharge tinged with blood and nagging thoughts about the biopsy threw me off balance. Embarrassed by the mix-up, I rummaged in a cluttered purse. *Don't tell me I forgot the checkbook!* After my gynecologist's associate completed the biopsy, I dressed quickly.

"I'll stop back by with the $15 co-pay," I promised the receptionist. I stepped out of the office and welcomed the invigorating blast of the cold night air. *Thank God that's over.* Just as I turned the key in the ignition, I noticed the doctor standing on the handicap ramp without a coat, waving frantically in my direction. *What did I forget now?* I wondered. At the touch of a button the window slid from view.

"Have you been taking iron?" she called.

"No."

"Then you need to," she admonished, disappearing in an instant. After a few minutes, she returned to the car with a hastily written prescription form. "You're probably anemic. This will help," she said as she shivered against the cold.

Like millions of women, I relied on a yearly pelvic exam and Pap test to monitor my reproductive health. It never occurred to me to check my symptoms against readily accessible information on the Internet or in my copy of the American Medical Association *Family Medical Guide.*

On Sunday, December 10, I approached the makeshift altar before worship service concluded. I joined several other worshippers who desired special prayer. Structural problems at the church's 160-year-old sanctuary had forced the congregation into temporary quarters. The Asbury United Methodist Church might not occupy a permanent church home, but that had not diminished the congregation's commitment to pray and serve with compassion. The Homestead Youth Association building housed the faithful this Sunday. Next week, the Camden Catholic High School cafeteria would welcome the worshipping flock. Like nomads wandering in the wilderness, we might not have a building, but we could pray.

"I'm waiting for the results of a biopsy. Pray with thanksgiving for God's healing," I whispered to Pastor Dennis Blackwell.

I waited for over a week for the pathologist's report.

Impatient for news of the results, I called the gynecologist's office on Monday, December 11, and again on Tuesday, to no avail.

"The lab's been swamped," the receptionist told me. "We'll call you."

Early Wednesday morning, despite the cold, I walked from home to a nearby lake. I carried one of several large rocks I keep on hand for such occasions. It was time to go "casting," a process by which a single rock represents my fears and cares. After identifying the menacing threat, I hurl that heavy burden as far into the lake as I can.

*Humble yourself under God's mighty hand, casting all your cares on Him. He cares for you (I Peter 5:7),* my Shepherd advised. Jesus Christ is the Shepherd and the Great Physician. He provided an important key before daybreak: *I will give you the treasures of darkness (Isaiah 45:3).* Walking to the lake with the rock in my right hand, I felt a surge of confidence. I belonged to God. He made me, and surely, He knew how to fix whatever was wrong. It might appear dark to me, but my mother had taught me long ago not to be governed by how things appear. If God said there were treasures of darkness and He'd give them to me, then so be it!

I threw that rock into the lake with a vengeance. I watched it arch and observed the ripple effects, the widening band of concentric circles after it splashed against the surface. Then I smiled. With the care for the biopsy results securely cast on the One who takes care, I experienced a peace that makes no sense at all, except *in the Spirit.*

# Chapter 2

## You Have Cancer

**For God hath not given us the spirit of fear; but of power, and of love, and of a sound mind. Be not thou therefore ashamed of the testimony of our Lord ...**

*II Timothy 1:7-8*

With only eleven days before Christmas, I didn't have time to waste. If I zipped into the gynecologist's office, paid the $15 fee for last week's office visit and biopsy, I'd be on my way in no time flat.

"I have my checkbook today," I said cheerfully, explaining the reason for the unexpected visit. I reached into my handbag and quickly located the little black book.

"We were just about to call you," the receptionist responded, obviously surprised to see me. "We have the biopsy results. Can you wait?" she asked.

I glanced at the clock: five minutes after ten o'clock. *Would* I wait? Had casting prepared me spiritually and emotionally to meet with the doctor alone?

"How long a wait?" I asked. Plenty of other things crowded today's agenda.

"Not very long. The doctor won't be long at all," she replied.

"Since I'm here, now *is* a good time," I agreed.

"Great ... Do you need to call work?" she asked.

"No. Not necessary," I responded quickly with a wave of the hand.

I shrugged off her suggestion as easily as I shrugged my shoulders. The freedom and flexibility of working for BTS Enterprises, Amos's advertising specialty company, was more precious than silver or gold. Hardworking, ambitious, and persistent, Amos had started a business providing customized imprinted merchandise and wearing apparel, and I helped him. Working part-time from our home's basement headquarters, he and I handled the administrative aspects of satisfying a wide range of clients. BTS offered everything from tee shirts or calculators for major corporations, to CD holders or jackets for area schools, to pens for political candidates, and utility knives for a local packaging store. You name it, and BTS could imprint it. It was a family affair, built with one satisfied client at a time over the past nine years. BTS: Better Trust the Savior. When Amos returned to full-time work as a software engineer four years ago, I single-handedly managed the business wearing a variety of hats from bookkeeper, marketing consultant, and graphic designer to delivery woman and janitor.

I sat down and casually observed the sassy Southwestern décor of the gynecologist's office. For the past five years, the warm terracotta, azure, and mauve hues invariably relaxed me. Three other women flipped disinterestedly through magazines. Only one made eye contact and smiled. I would not wait long. This had the distinct feel of a divine appointment. It certainly wasn't on my schedule. The result of the endometrial biopsy was out of my control. After another busy week since the doctor performed the biopsy, God had me in the right place: the waiting room.

In less than ten minutes, the doctor's nursing assistant called my name and ushered me into an exam room. Replete with a large potted plant, an oversized basket full of dog-eared magazines, a cushioned wicker chair, and the whimsical touch of hot pink socks covering the stirrups on the examination table, the room afforded a cozy setting for uncomfortable situations. This was the first gynecologist I ever visited who showed compassion by warming the speculum before conducting the pelvic exam.

Stylishly dressed in a black pantsuit, Dr. Stanley entered the exam room around half past ten.

"Hi, Doc," I said cheerfully.

"The news is not good," she said soberly.

The great shield of faith deflected the blow. I had both asked and thanked the Great Physician for healing me nearly two weeks ago. I had the key.

*I am healed. My faith has made me whole.*

I nodded for her to proceed.

"You have cancer of the uterus," she declared solemnly.

I heard the words, but steadfast and immovable, I spoke calmly.

"What did the biopsy show?" I asked in a measured tone, unblinking as I maintained direct eye contact.

I detected trepidation in Dr. Stanley's eyes and a distinct heaviness in her usually buoyant bearing as she delivered the sad news that Thursday morning. Little did I know she also carefully measured my response. Holding the pathologist's report in hand, she pointed to the text: endometrial adenocarcinoma. The biopsy found this slow-growing cancer invading my most intimate parts.

"You will need a hysterectomy right away," she intoned with precision and urgency.

I nodded again, still calibrating her gaze.

"I've taken the liberty of referring you to a gynecological oncologist. We have scheduled an appointment for 3:45 this afternoon. Do you think you can make it?" she concluded.

Having outlined the diagnosis, treatment, and the direction for *my* next step, she relaxed her professional demeanor and awaited my reaction. Would I weep with anguished sobs or cry with uncontrollable sorrow? Would I sit in silent shock or rigid denial? She seemed to brace herself . . . preparing to both comfort and console, or to restate the medical case, if necessary. At the time, I did not believe she had the slightest clue to my response.

"Where is the oncologist located?" I asked simply. After all, healing requires faithful commitment to the next step in the process of change . . . whatever it is. The specialist's location was important because *my* next step, the next thing on the "to do" list involved BTS business, a scheduled tee shirt delivery to one of my high school clients. If I planned to make a late-afternoon doctor's appointment, I'd better get going.

"He's right here in town. I'll get his card," she replied. "You seem to be taking this very well," she added.

Nodding slightly, I now smiled. "God is with me. I know He didn't bring me this far to leave me," I affirmed with faithful confidence. Whatever lay ahead, God knew about it, had made provision for it, and I wasn't ashamed to say it.

The diagnosis did not paralyze me with fear because I had a key: I belong to God.

Dr. Stanley left the exam room. Obviously relieved to conclude our time together, she needed no formality now. With business concluded, I collected my coat and handbag and left the exam room too. From my vantage point in the corridor, I saw her rummaging through a cluttered drawer with uncharacteristic agitation.

"Here's his card," she said. She handed me an ink-stained, crumpled business card.

*When was the last time she referred this guy?*

For the moment I could leave with everything I needed well in hand.

"Let us know how things work out. You're going to be okay," she assured me, patting my hand. "Keep us posted."

When I entered the waiting room area, the receptionist reached across her desk to squeeze my hand. She wished me luck.

"Thanks," I said, pressing my lips with resolve.

The lucky ones can only thank their lucky stars. As for me, I left Dr. Stanley's office thanking God. Deep within my inner self, God's peace flooded my soul. To the human eye it looked like I was walking, but *in the Spirit* I was leaping and hopping and praising God! I AM healed of any fear, despair, or hopelessness concerning the biopsy results, the diagnosis, or the proposed treatment. *I have life and peace!*

# Chapter 3

## Conflicting Diagnoses

**For God is not the author of confusion, but of peace . . .**

*I Corinthians 14:33*

I entered the midmorning traffic headed northbound on Route 295 toward Trenton and quickly accelerated to sixty-five miles per hour. Turning up the volume on the smooth jazz station, I laughed out loud.

"I could get creamed by one of these eighteen-wheelers," I chuckled. "No need to worry about cancer," I concluded with customary logic. It wasn't quite eleven o'clock. That would allow time to deliver the shirts, eat lunch, and still be on time for the 3:45 appointment with the gynecological oncologist referred by Dr. Stanley.

Breezing southbound down the highway headed home, I felt relieved. With the delivery accomplished and another client satisfied, I needed to talk with Amos. Once inside the front door, I reached for the telephone. Hearing his voice on the answering machine was disappointing. *I couldn't very well leave that message,* I thought with a wry smile.

Let's see. Thursday . . . Dana's art lesson started after school at four o'clock. *I need someone to drive her over there, Lord.* There's always something to do next, I mused. *How did people get bored anyway,* I wondered.

"Hi . . . It's Irene. Can you take Dana to art lessons this afternoon?"

"Sure, no problem," my neighbor Donna readily agreed.

"I have a doctor's appointment this afternoon, and I really appreciate it," I explained.

"I'll pick her up at about ten minutes to four. Don't worry about it," she said.

Grateful that only one call sufficed for Dana's transportation arrangements, I hung up and prepared to dial again.

I needed specific directions to the doctor's office. Looking at the ink-stained business card, I shook my head.

*When **was** the last time she referred this guy, Lord?*

I dialed but reached the wrong number. Absently thinking I had dialed incorrectly, I tried again. After all, I had a lot on my mind. A few seconds after the second unsuccessful try, the phone rang while still in my hand. Startled, I pressed the "on" button.

"May I speak to Irene Pace?"

"This is Irene."

"This is the doctor's office calling to confirm your 3:45 appointment this afternoon."

*Well, what do you know!* I requested directions and asked the woman to confirm the phone number. The number on the card was incorrect.

*You're in this, Lord. I know it.*

I dialed Amos again, but still no answer. As the phone rang in my ear, I suddenly remembered his standing two o'clock Thursday meeting. A senior engineer at Lockheed Martin, he was probably at lunch and wouldn't be free until after four o'clock, at least. With all that had happened this morning, I'd completely forgotten.

Since the oncologist's office was only a fifteen-minute drive from home, I sat in the living room to collect my thoughts before the next thing beckoned. Seated on the sofa opposite the big picture window, I looked out on towering pines, stately in silhouette against a clear blue sky. This year, our Christmas tree graced the corner opposite the vaulted ceiling. I liked the balance it gave the rectangular room. Fresh cut from a neighbor's lakefront property, the tree's fragrant aroma brought back warm memories of Christmas past. I tarried only briefly on holiday recollections. The impact of the day's events overshadowed all other thoughts.

"She said I had cancer . . ."

*Thank you, Lord, for healing me!*

God had already healed my mind back in 1980, so I knew He could heal my body. God removed the guilt and shame that had settled over me like a wet, moldy blanket. Today I remembered and thanked Him.

I located the doctor's office easily with time to spare for calm reflection. I sat in the parked car for about ten minutes.

*Thank you, Lord, for loving me!*

Today I connected the dots of God's merciful intervention and amazing grace in many impossible situations before this present moment. I remembered driving in blinding fog. I remembered when Amos and I didn't have two nickels between us. I remembered the day Lorraine came into the world. I remembered how God orchestrated events the day Dana was born. Today I remembered and thanked the Lord.

When I entered the office, the sign-in sheet affixed to a clipboard provided a poor substitute for a warm, friendly greeting. Bold print at the bottom of the page offered the only direction: please take a seat. The offices appeared to be empty. I supposed *someone* would help me shortly. I glanced around and noticed a few chairs to the right down a wide sloping hallway. I perched on the edge of the chair and looked around. On one side of a wide hallway, I saw three closed doors with wall racks for patient charts. On the other side of the hall, rows of framed caricatures lined the wall and continued into an adjoining room. The portraits covered nearly every square inch of available wall space. I walked around regarding the drawings with amused interest. They reminded me of those hastily sketched five-minute portraits sold by boardwalk artists.

When I returned to my seat, I noticed a wall collage of thoughtful letters and carefully chosen cards from patients and family members thanking the doctor for his care. I stood to read them.

"Thanks so much for your compassion . . ."

"Now that Mom has passed . . ."

"You were so kind during the difficult last days . . ."

I immediately stopped reading and gulped. The visual image of the words on paper stung my eyes. Blinking, I shook my head as if to clear my brain of some annoying cobweb. The distinctive collage melted all courage like butter on a hot potato. *Better drop it!* I immediately plopped back into the chair. In one continuous motion, I swept my black wool coat over crossed knees, folded my arms, and waited. That was enough of that. I wanted to live.

*What am I doing here, Lord? What's going on? Where is everybody? Anybody? I sure wish Amos was here.*

The caricatures regained their bizarre appeal. I stood again to survey the distorted faces attached to disproportioned bodies. About ten minutes later, a nurse appeared.

"The doctor will be with you very soon," she said with a smile.

A few minutes later, a man emerged from one of the closed doors. Dressed in black slacks, a black V-neck sweater and white turtleneck, he rounded the corner with speed and purpose. Of medium build, he looked to be in his early forties.

"Someone will be right with you," he said in a high-pitched, cheery voice. He walked quickly toward the front entrance and stopped near the sign-up sheet. He reminded me of the Mad Hatter, only he wore a black skullcap. An overweight woman who looked to be in her late sixties and a tired-looking man shuffled along shortly after the energetic one. The elderly gentleman extended his hand and thanked the younger man profusely.

"I'll see you in two weeks," the shrill voice reminded.

*Was that the doctor, Lord? Since Amos isn't here, I'm sure glad you're with me, Father.*

A short time later, a woman dressed in a print smock blouse called my name and requested insurance information.

*I praise your name, Lord, for providing health insurance. Just a few months ago, when Amos was laid off for three months, I didn't have this card, Jesus.*

She ushered me into a very large examination room. The exam table with its narrow strip of white paper sat to the right. A silver gooseneck floor lamp stood like a sentry near the stirrups. Three white plastic chairs rested alone on the far-left wall. Painted a nondescript bluish gray, the room, both cold and sterile, contrasted sharply with the warm and cozy atmosphere in my gynecologist's office. No socks on the stirrups this time. After taking a preliminary history, the nurse left me alone.

*Well . . . here I am.* Sure, I'd thought about breast cancer. Who practices monthly self breast exams on two normal breasts without thinking about the possibility of disease? But who would have imagined I'd develop cancer of the uterus after faithfully undergoing an annual pelvic exam and Pap test for the past twenty-five years?

I pulled the fax copy of the pathologist's report from my portfolio. *Adenocarcinoma.* I winced at the sound of the word. Unfortunately, I was completely ignorant about the limitations of the Pap test as a screening test for cancer. It is not a diagnostic test. Year after year, I felt relieved and breathed easily until the next exam, but I was uninformed. A positive Pap test result *can* warn a woman that something may be wrong, but a negative result *cannot* assure her that everything is all right, especially if there is a history of multiple sexual partners.

*Well . . . here I am, Lord. It's just you and me. Too bad I couldn't reach Amos.*

A light knock on the door signaled the doctor's arrival. He energetically entered the room and extended his hand in greeting.

"So tell me what's been happening," he said, pulling up a rolling stool.

I looked squarely in his eyes, took a deep breath, and recounted the specific details. I told him about the onset of the watery discharge tinged with blood the first Friday in November while visiting my daughter at Cornell. I mentioned the start of my regular period the following Monday and added the normal flow stopped five days later as it had since I was thirteen years old. I talked about the initial visit to the gynecologist on November 16 after my period stopped and the discharge continued. I remembered to tell him about using the five-day supply of metronidazole gel, the messy vaginal suppository prescribed after the initial pelvic exam. I became animated for a moment and related how I was usually pretty energetic, but over the past few weeks a chronic tiredness seemed to have settled into my weary bones. I told him about the endometrial biopsy on December 5 and that I'd just received the results today: the tissue sample showed cancer of the uterus. I exhaled, and I handed him the pathologist's report. The oncologist listened intently and took some notes during my discourse. He looked carefully over the printed facsimile page, and then he spoke.

"I'm going to need to examine you, and then we can talk further," he said.

*Here we go, Lord. You know I hate this part.*

As if on cue, the doctor left the room, and the nurse appeared.

"Take off everything from the waist down," she directed as she handed me a disposable cloth sheet.

I wrapped the stiff fabric around my torso and sat stiffly on the exam table. Nervous, I fully reclined and stared at the white ceiling.

*Here I am, Lord.*

The nurse returned first and rolled a table into view with protective rubber gloves for the doctor, a tube of lubricating gel, and a stainless steel speculum. The doctor entered and clicked the light switch. The exam had begun. After I dutifully scooted to the end of the table, the nurse adjusted my heels in the stirrups. The gynecological oncologist probed deeply and aggressively during the exam. As a mother of two, I'd had many pelvic exams before, but no one had ever placed fingers in the vagina and the rectum at the same time. Probing, extending fingers touched the left and right perimetrium, the tissues surrounding the reproductive organs. The painful investigation of my intimate anatomy seemed so humiliating. Immodestly draped, I felt utterly violated. During the exam, he dictated exam notes in a strident, professional cadence. As required by law, his nurse was present, but that didn't change my sense of vulnerability and victimization.

"Do you have to probe so deeply?" I asked, visibly shaken and squirming beneath the stiff white covering.

"I don't mean to hurt you," he replied with compassion and professionalism. "I need to check you as thoroughly as possible."

Lying on that table, I recalled the horrible time when I was the victim of date rape during spring break of my junior year in college. Totally traumatized, I felt so violated and ashamed that day. No, I never reported the shameful incident nearly thirty years ago. I just showered like there was no tomorrow and cried a river of tears while the warm water flowed. No, I was not a victim today, not even a cancer victim. Today, I was a new patient seeing a cancer specialist, a male gynecological oncologist referred by a female gynecologist. This was radically different from being a scared college coed trapped in a bad relationship that led to a criminal act. Nonetheless, I felt the same. The door to a response other than guilt, shame, and wanting to die seemed closed at that moment. Closed, until I heard the Shepherd's voice.

*Use your mind to serve me. I've set you free. That was then, and this is now. There is therefore now no condemnation to those who belong to Christ Jesus and follow the Spirit. All is forgiven. I've told you repeatedly: You are mine, and I love you. This is the key. There is no condemnation now.*

Struggling up on one elbow, I collected myself and wrapped the paper sheet around me.

"What did you find?" I immediately wanted to know.

"Why don't you get dressed first, then we'll talk about it," he replied, snapping the inverted rubber glove from his hand.

I moved very slowly.

*Help me, Lord . . . I need you to help me. I cannot do this.*

Once again, it was not an audible voice, yet I heard the words clearly. In a spirit of peace, I dressed quickly and gathered my belongings. *No condemnation.* I'd be leaving soon, headed home and into Amos's arms. *I am loved.* I'd get a second opinion at the Hospital of the University of Pennsylvania (HUP) where I had worked as a volunteer. I had options.

*I am free. Thank you, Holy Spirit. I'm holding on.*

I left the exam room, and the nurse directed me to the doctor's office for consultation. I found the oncologist seated behind a small desk with an open pharmaceutical manual illustrating the female reproductive organs.

"Based on my exam, you have stage IIB cervical cancer, not endometrial cancer," he pronounced with confidence. "There is perimetrial extension on the left side," he continued, pointing to the diagram.

"Can you explain that, Doctor?" I asked.

Using his ink pen, he identified specific areas of the female reproductive system. I sighed and listened.

*To be spiritually minded is life and peace. Keep your focus on me, Irene.*

I used a key: *He will keep him in perfect peace whose mind is stayed on thee.*

"How is this treated?" I asked.

"We'll need to get a CT scan of the pelvis, and you'll need chemotherapy and radiation to begin immediately," he explained.

"Two years ago, I was a volunteer at the Hospital of the University of Pennsylvania working with cancer patients. I still have some contacts, and I'll be seeking a second opinion there," I responded.

The oncologist presented a case for the cancer treatment center with which he was affiliated. He strongly suggested I not delay treatment and asked if I would consent to having some blood work done before leaving. He suspected iron deficiency anemia, especially since I'd been losing blood. Low hemoglobin levels would also account for increasing fatigue. The prescription drug Procrit would help produce the necessary red blood cells to carry oxygen from the lungs to the body's other cells. Procrit would also help when the chemotherapy started, he explained.

*Lord, this is all happening so fast. What should I do?*

It is hard to explain why I didn't thank him and leave the office right then and there. I knew I would get a second opinion, but I did not resist his urgent suggestion for blood work because my energy level had declined so precipitously since Thanksgiving.

"Just one question, Doc," I asked, after agreeing to stay for the blood tests. "If your wife presented with this condition, where would you want her treated?"

*Did he say HUP, Lord?*

The blood work took only a few minutes, but I waited over an hour for the test results and the administration of the forty thousand units of Procrit. My hemoglobin count was 9.7. A count from 12.0 to 18.0 is considered in the normal reference range. As I leafed through outdated magazines, I remembered a visit to these offices about four years ago on another referral for iron deficiency anemia. I remembered careening from the parking lot that day. I left with a distinct impression: they think I have cancer!

Today, the nurse ushered me into a large room with a dozen reclining chairs. She took a blood pressure reading, and then generously swabbed the skin on my upper right arm. Next, she swiftly plunged a hypodermic needle into a small vial.

"This is going to sting," she said, before sinking the needle into my arm.

*Jesus! Lord Jesus!*

The painful injection created a burning sensation like a cattle brand. Though tightly closed, my eyes rolled as the full thrust of the fiery, stinging medication flowed into my veins. The nurse rubbed the burning arm with a gloved hand.

"I know that hurts. It's going to pass," she said consolingly. "You'll be okay."

I collected my belongings for the last time. It was later than I thought. No one sat at the desk to request the $15 co-pay. Bright halogen lights illuminated the parking lot pathway. As I drove away, I rubbed the sore arm again. My thoughts drifted to a friend, a cervical cancer survivor, who would understand how exhausted and dehumanized I felt. We had talked, prayed often, and even laughed together during her illness and recovery. While others might understand, Amos took first place.

*Help me, Holy Spirit, to tell my husband the awful news.*

# Part II

## Waters, Floods and Fire

# Chapter 4

## Lead Balloons

☞ Fear them not . . . for there is nothing covered that shall not be revealed; and hid, that shall not be known.

*Matthew 10:26*

Turning left into our suburban development, I thanked God for bringing me safely back to our tree-lined lane once more. After thirteen years at the same address, I refused to take safe travels for granted. With two minor car accidents on my driving record, I drove with care, respectful and wary of New Jersey's astronomical automobile insurance rates. The automatic garage door opened to reveal a motley assortment of shelves filled with years of collected clutter. Home at last, I found Amos seated at the kitchen table opening the day's mail.

"Hi, doll," he greeted me with outstretched arms. "How's my peaches?"

I smiled, acknowledging his fondness for various terms of endearment. Since he was seated, I moved to plant a quick arms-around-his-neck hug. Instead, he stood to embrace me warmly.

"I need a real hug," he said.

"Me too."

"I love you today."

"I love you every day."

"How did things go today? Did you get out to the school with the shirts?"

I stepped out of his embrace. The pleasantries ended far too soon. He returned to sort mail and absently started to ask questions. I slipped my coat off weary shoulders.

"So, did they like the shirts?"

"Yeah," I responded absently. "I've had a full plate today. Where's Dana?" I asked, changing the subject.

"She's upstairs doing her homework. Did you get in touch with the doctor?"

I nodded, sighed, and sat across the table from him. Wrinkles rippled across his forehead.

*Help me, Lord Jesus.*

"I saw the doctor this morning. I tried to call you several times. She said I had cancer."

Amos's face registered shock and disbelief. He didn't speak for several moments. The furrows deepened in his brow. Tears welled in my eyes and his.

"Is she sure? How does she know for sure?" he asked at last in rapid-fire succession. I reached across the table to grasp his hand.

"The biopsy, honey. I saw a specialist this afternoon. The pathology report showed cancer. Adenocarcinoma."

It was a difficult, cumbersome word, as heavy as a lead balloon.

*Help us, Holy Ghost.*

Neither one of us spoke. We simply sat, just staring into each other's tear-filled eyes. Amos finally broke the tearful silence.

"How are you doing? Are you all right?"

I could not speak.

"I've failed you. I feel like I've failed you," he repeated in anguish.

"Honey? What are you talking about? No. No, you haven't failed me. You love me," I affirmed and squeezed his hand. "You didn't give me cancer. Look . . . God is in this. Just like He's always been."

He reached into his back pocket for a folded handkerchief and wiped his eyes.

"Let's pray," he said. We bowed our heads in unison.

Amos extended strong arms across the table. Our outstretched arms formed parallel lines as we clasped each other's hands. When Amos finished praying, I knew there were obstacles ahead, but *cancer* didn't stand a chance.

"So tell me what happened," he said as he settled back into his chair. He absently massaged his temples. With both hands, he slowly pulled downward across his eyes and nose.

I recounted the specific details of the conversation with Dr. Stanley and the conflict in the diagnosis based on the oncologist's findings. I told him how humiliated I felt during the pelvic examination. I was just about to mention the low blood count and the Procrit injection, when Dana bounded downstairs, checked her reflection in the foyer mirror, and entered the kitchen.

"Hi, Mom, what's for dinner?" she asked, opening the refrigerator for a can of soda.

Our private time was over.

"Is everything okay? You guys don't look too good. What's wrong?" Dana asked perceptively.

"We're okay," I lied. "Did you get to your art lesson all right?" I asked, changing the subject for the second time tonight. I wasn't ready to tell Dana yet. *I'll wait until Saturday when Lorraine comes home and tell them both at the same time,* I thought. Kill two birds with one stone.

*Help me, Lord Jesus.*

"How's your painting coming?" I asked. "How's Lisa?" I inquired about my friend, the neighborhood art teacher.

"She's good. Are you all right Mom? You look so tired."

"Just a really busy day," I replied.

Dana looked skeptical. "I'm going up to finish my homework."

Sighing heavily, I started dinner preparations. Not surprisingly, I wasn't very hungry. Thank God for leftovers. I quickly calculated the untold benefit of moving quickly past this juncture of the journey. There was simply too much to do and too little time.

Lorraine's final exams ended the next day. Amos and I needed to finalize arrangements for the Saturday morning drive to transport Lorraine and all her gear safely back home. For Thanksgiving break, she settled for a scheduled six-hour bus ride through Manhattan's Port Authority with plans to arrive at a bus station only ten minutes from home. Unfortunately, the trip stretched into a grueling nine-hour fiasco with a drive to the bus depot in Philadelphia to boot! For Christmas break, she asked for mercy rather than risk another marathon bus ride during the peak holiday season. Dana and I had work to do, so Amos planned to drive to Cornell alone. I was uncomfortable.

"Have you thought about calling anybody to make the trip with you? You've already had a full week at work, now this is on your mind, and you're tired. Did you ask your brother?" I badgered. "I just don't want you making that long drive by yourself."

"Broxie didn't get back to me yet," he replied absently in reference to my brother-in-law.

"What about Bruce?" I asked, mentally searching for someone, anyone who lived nearby, who might be available Saturday morning.

"That's an idea. I'll give him a call tonight."

Amos gathered the mail. After thanking God for the food, the three of us ate in relative silence.

"So are you looking forward to your sister coming back home?" I asked Dana between bites of chicken salad. Lorraine's winter break lasted five weeks.

"Yeah. But I'm not too excited about sharing my bathroom."

After Dana excused herself from the table to finish homework, Amos and I spent a long time talking in the kitchen. A somber mood settled over the table strewn with empty bowls and dirty plates. Darkness seemed to infiltrate other rooms too. When we finally retired to our bedroom, we spoke very little. Exhausted and heavy-hearted, we lay silently in bed propped on pillows. Then, Amos called Dana into the room.

"Am I in trouble?"

"You always say that, Dana," I chuckled. "No, you're not in any trouble."

"Is something wrong?"

In a soft voice I told my daughter the truth: "I went to the doctor this morning, honey. She said I had cancer."

Dana's eyes locked on mine, but she kept her distance.

"Mom? Are you all right?"

I wanted to hug Dana and shield her from the weight of this awful news, but she so rarely returned my embrace.

"I'll be going to HUP for a second opinion, honey. There was some confusion regarding the diagnosis," I explained. "My regular gynecologist said I had uterine cancer, but I saw a specialist this afternoon, and he said it was cervical cancer. So I have to get things straightened out. That's the first step," I assured my teenage daughter.

While I spoke, Dana stood fixed as if there was an invisible wooden barrier between us. She needed space.

"Is it hereditary?" she asked insightfully.

I deeply respected her immediate need to create even more distance between us.

"What's going to happen to you, Mom?"

"God has this, honey. I have His Word on it," I replied. "I've prayed. Your dad prayed. Our God hears and answers with power," I reassured us both.

Amos led the prayers once more. Dana bowed her head, but she didn't break down and cry. After goodnight hugs and kisses, she left the room. Under the cover of darkness I rolled to one side and curled into a ball. Like Dana, I shed no public tears. Yet, the weight of the cancer diagnosis inflicted enough pain to make a grown man cry.

In nearly twenty-six years of marriage, I could count the times I'd seen tears in my husband's eyes. He cried when his older brother died suddenly following an epileptic seizure. John, a decorated Vietnam War veteran, had started having attacks after taking shrapnel from a mortar shell. After returning home, he was continuously plagued with convulsive seizures. Alcohol consumption seemed to transform him from Dr. Jekyll into Mr. Hyde. John died at age thirty-eight. My mother-in-law called to tell Amos the regrettable news. With silent tears, he repeated the conversation. We lived in Rhode Island then, and he made the six-hour drive to Chester alone in a record three and a half hours.

Tears blurred his vision a second time when his father passed away. After returning from the funeral home in final preparation for the viewing and burial, Amos expressed profound sadness.

"He looked like an African king. Like royalty," he recounted as his eyes filled up. I never heard audible sobbing, just simple silent tears like the ones clouding his eyes tonight. My father-in-law suffered from the ravages of alcoholism all the years I knew him. Liver complications took their eventual toll on his health. He was a hardworking, hard-drinking brick mason and contractor; his ten children had the same mother. He remained married for nearly fifty years, until his death.

*All tears associated with death and dying*, I thought sadly.

Then, I remembered the very last time I'd seen Amos cry. He shed tears of joy at the conclusion of *It's a Wonderful Life*, the movie classic where Jimmy Stewart's character realizes the man who has friends is the richest man in town. Amos is such a man.

The middle son of ten children, Amos grew up literally fighting his way through childhood and adolescence on Chester's mean streets. With no hope or plan to attend college, he looked to the region's major employer, the Scott Paper Company, for what he thought would be a lifetime of factory work after finishing high school in 1970. But God had a different plan. One year shy of the required age for employment, he was turned down by Scott Paper.

"Come back next year," they told him.

This timely rejection at age seventeen turned out to be a blessing in disguise. During the summer after graduation, recruiters from DeVry Institute of Technology canvassed his neighborhood. Amos jumped at the chance to move to Chicago. By the time we met in December 1971, he had nearly completed requirements for a two-year associate's degree in electronic technology while holding down two jobs.

One night-shift job landed him on the ninety-seventh floor of Chicago's John Hancock Building. The elevated train ride from Northwestern University's Evanston campus took nearly an hour. Awed by the spectacular views of the city's sprawling southern and western expanses, and the vastness of Lake Michigan to the east, I visited him regularly on the weekends. We studied some. We also talked about our families and envisioned bright futures that would shine like the noonday sun. Amos wanted to earn an electrical engineering degree, return to Chester, and help his family. His vision involved improving the impoverished community where he was raised. My goals involved completion of a journalism degree at Northwestern. I wanted to become a newspaper reporter and also write compelling fiction books filled with unforgettable characters like those I knew from childhood. Barely twenty years old, our hopes and dreams shimmered and shined like the city's dazzling night-lights that glowed beneath us from our private ninety-seventh-floor observatory. We formed a strong friendship, fell in love, and married three years later in December 1974. Now, almost twenty-six years to the day we said "I do," life and all its challenges just kept coming. Lots of water accumulated under the bridge in all those years, but we were still standing on God's promise to keep us together, come what may. We might be seasoned married folks, but this cancer hurdle placed us squarely in the infancy of something we'd never faced before.

The next morning, I received a call from the oncologist's office. The doctor wanted me to schedule a CT scan of the pelvis, a routine diagnostic imaging test that would confirm the diagnosis, and a chest X-ray to detect potential spread of disease. The friendly voice informed me she had taken the liberty of setting up appointments for these procedures at a local radiology center one week later on Friday, December 22. The oncologist also wanted me to come in Monday morning to discuss any questions and sign the release forms to start chemotherapy.

*They've taken a lot of liberties here, Father God.*

I wanted clarity on the diagnosis before proceeding further. So did Amos. I definitely planned to get a second opinion from HUP, although I had yet to call.

I agreed to the CT scan and X-ray but deferred on the Monday appointment until after I spoke with Amos.

As soon as the conversation ended, I dialed Amos's number.

"The oncologist wants me to come in on Monday to sign off on the chemo," I told Amos. "He'll be there to answer our questions."

"I want to meet this guy, but you won't be signing anything," he replied.

Next, I called the office of Dr. David Zalut, my primary care physician, to arrange for the necessary electronic referrals for the two procedures. Office policy required at least two days advance notice to process a referral, so I had some time. But Christmas Day was right around the corner.

I also called a friend who might provide some answers, even though we had not spoken in nearly two years. Still, I looked up her number in my phone book with confidence. If I reached out to discuss cancer, I knew she would respond. To my surprise and consternation, her number was not in the book.

"Oh, for crying out loud," I complained. "Who can believe this? Where's her number?"

The next second . . . no, in less than a second, the once-familiar number just popped into my head, and I dialed it. A recorded message announced the number had changed. The nasal voice of the operator enunciated the new listing, but the area code was not in New Jersey. Believing God knows all things, I dialed again.

A woman said "hello." I instantly recognized her very sleepy voice.

"Hi! This is Irene Pace."

"I don't believe it. How are you?"

"Did I wake you?"

"It's okay. I needed to get up anyway. How are the girls?"

I provided a brief update on the girls' activities, including Lorraine's scheduled arrival the next day and Dana's artistic success. It was just like old times, chatting back and forth. A busy working mother, she didn't have any time to waste either. I got right to the point.

"I needed to talk with you because I've been diagnosed with cancer, but there's some confusion regarding the diagnosis."

There was a long pause. "Are you okay? Did you get a second opinion yet?"

"I'm okay with it. Remember the day you called to tell me about your diagnosis? It's like that. God's got this."

"Yeah, I do remember. I want to see you. I'm free all of next week. What's good for you?"

I mentioned the appointment with the oncologist Monday morning. We agreed to meet at my house at noon.

"Just don't sign anything," she admonished.

The weekend schedule and bookings into next week were filling up fast that Friday morning, and it wasn't even ten o'clock yet. I needed to tackle the never-ending stack of BTS paperwork and go to the grocery store. I hoped to close the office the Wednesday before Christmas. Taking an indefinite leave of absence sounded like a great idea.

Amos and Bruce left for Ithaca shortly after eight o'clock Saturday morning. By the time Amos returned with Lorraine, Dana and I had trimmed the tree, decked the halls, cleaned the house, cooked lasagna, baked brownies, prepared a salad, set the table, and started a roaring blaze in the family room fireplace. All the while, we chimed in with the "Hallelujah Chorus" turned full blast on the CD player and sang along to some of our favorite holiday and R and B tunes. It was a lot of work, but we truly had fun working together.

They said "I had cancer," but it was Christmas, for heaven's sake. I wanted Lorraine and Amos to find the familiar festive atmosphere I loved to create this time of year. No two years were ever alike. By the second week of December, plans to "make Christmas," whatever the budget for holiday decorations, were typically in high gear. From setting up an elaborate manger that once belonged to my mother to festooning the banister from the foyer to the upstairs hall, I rejoiced to know this Christ and Son. For me, Jesus is the reason for the season.

"Did you tell Lorraine?" I whispered to Amos before we started dinner.

"I thought you should tell her," he replied.

After dinner, Lorraine and I ventured downstairs to enjoy hot chocolate and dessert by the warmth of the fire. Quite naturally, we talked about Cornell and her adjustment to college life. A computer science major, Lorraine carried a full load during the fall semester including courses in computer science, cognitive science, calculus, and the required freshman writing seminar. She had even taken a sailing course that ended right before Thanksgiving. Call it mother's intuition: she needed a break.

"So how did your exams go?"

"They're over. Thank God," she said, sounding truly relieved. She mentioned the names of new friends in her dorm and shared some of their exploits.

"Any special young men in your life up there?" I inquired in motherly fashion. Her easy laughter and laid-back style refreshed me. I enjoyed a comfortable relationship with my daughter. She had matured in perceptible ways since that long-ago day back in August when we loaded a truckload of her gear into a rented minivan. Quite honestly, I preferred not to interject a heavy lead balloon into our conversation, but she had to be told.

"Did your dad tell you I'd been to the doctor?"

"No, what's up?"

I swallowed hard. "I've been diagnosed with cancer, Lorraine."

"Oh, Mom. Mom."

*Mom.* A low baleful moan seemed to echo from within Lorraine's inner core. The reverberations shattered my own fragile psyche. Instinctively, we reached out to one another and hugged tightly. For several moments we were so closely knit I could taste the sharp, biting twinge of her sorrow. The heaviness suffocated momentarily, but I refused to hold it. Tears welled up in both our eyes, but only a few spilled out. We swallowed the rest.

"Are you okay, Mom? Are you going to be okay?"

"I'm healed, honey. I've asked God to heal me."

"What happened? How did you find out?"

I told her about the onset of the discharge and the subsequent biopsy.

"Why didn't you tell me? Even at Thanksgiving, you didn't tell me," she accused.

"I didn't want you to worry. Besides, I didn't know anything then. I just found out on Thursday, and I wasn't going to tell you over the phone," I defended. "Besides, I'm going to get a second opinion."

"At HUP?"

I nodded in assent, although I still had not called the hospital. "People will be praying for me there. In all likelihood, I will be treated there." *On Monday, I'll call on Monday*, I silently promised.

Now that Lorraine knew the situation, I felt like four bombshells had dropped in three days. Dodging the shrapnel took skill and precision. First, I got hit, but thank God for the shield of faith. Then, I quickly discovered it wasn't any easier to tell the people I loved what doctors reported than it was for my loved ones to hear it. The words 'you have cancer' can strike with the fury of an undetected missile. The lightning flash can blind and debilitate even the most stout-hearted optimist. It is painfully difficult news both to hear and to tell.

I sat in silence with my daughter and held her hand. The glowing fire gave the family room a comfortable ambience, but this wasn't some made-for-TV movie that would end in time for the eleven o'clock news. This was my life on the line. But I was choosing life, no matter what "they" said. If it meant climbing uphill, so be it. I had a Shepherd to lead the way. I'd seen Him make a way out of no way before. My circumstances had changed, but He was the same.

*Thank you, Lord, for healing me and helping my family through this.*

I immediately made up my mind to agree with God. The Bible says, *"There's nothing hidden that won't be revealed."* Therefore, I decided to inform a wide circle of family members, friends, and neighbors, starting tomorrow. My reasoning was simple: if faithful people knew the truth regarding my health status and *prayed*, then God would answer these intercessory prayers with power, just like He promised.

*God is looking to show himself strong on my behalf.*

At worship service the next morning in the high school cafeteria, I approached the altar without hesitation when Pastor Blackwell asked if anyone needed prayer. Amos and the girls followed. The four of us held hands at the altar.

"Irene's been diagnosed with cancer, Pastor," Amos whispered.

"Please pray with thanksgiving," I whispered with insistence.

With my back to the congregation, I heard gasps when Pastor Blackwell announced the diagnosis. In an outpouring of love and with overwhelming tenderness, the congregation showed support and compassion. Many believers came forward to stand with us at the altar. By the time Pastor Blackwell finished praying, there was hardly a dry eye in the place, mine included.

"Pray with thanksgiving," I told everyone as we embraced. There were hugs all around . . . tight, heartfelt hugs and warm, tender embraces for my family and me. The faithful affirmed God's healing power, and it deeply encouraged my heart that Sunday morning. I drew considerable strength from many at the altar who were cancer survivors themselves. They had firsthand experience with God's power to heal hearts, minds, and bodies. I received the blessings, prayers, and testimonies of these eyewitnesses with genuine gladness and profound gratitude.

After worship service, I started making phone calls: first, to Dad in Chicago and then to my sister Susan in Denver. I also called another woman I've known since childhood days. These were the first of many conversations to break the silence and solicit prayers with thanksgiving. In a few short days, God heard fervent prayers from around the country . . . petitions from a community of believers committed to ask God to help me. Later Sunday evening, I dusted off the medical reference guide, while Amos surfed the Internet for various cancer sites and showed me his findings.

I read the big bold print in utter disbelief. A watery vaginal discharge tinged with blood is one of the primary symptoms of cancer of the cervix or uterus. No one told me. I didn't know. No one mentioned the human papilloma virus (HPV) either. HPV is a sexually transmitted disease. Infection with HPV is the primary risk factor for cervical cancer. More than 75 percent of sexually active men and women have been exposed to the virus. Certain strains of HPV result in a highly contagious infection that can cause the eruption of vaginal and/or cervical warts. Other risk factors include having sexual intercourse with multiple partners, who also have multiple partners, and commencing sexual intercourse at an early age before the sensitive cervical area fully develops. I was stunned.

I opened the door to disease a few weeks before my nineteenth birthday in the closing days of freshman year in college. Unwanted pregnancy was the greatest fear. To be honest, I never gave STD's more than a passing thought until doctors treated awful, itchy warts during sophomore year. After that, I reassessed my life. The warts never returned and I had no other incidences of an STD. No one told me about HPV and its link to cervical cancer at the university infirmary or *anytime* after that, even during all the recent pelvic examinations.

Now, I stared at the computer screen in total shock. A World Health Organization (WHO) report pulled no punches: "Infection with HPV usually occurs in the early years of sexual activity, but it takes up to 20 years to develop into a malignant tumor." The organization called cervical cancer a sexually transmitted disease caused by HPV. Scientists believe essentially all cervical cancer is caused by infection with two high-risk strains of the nearly one hundred known human papilloma viruses. WHO researchers discovered the HPV trigger in 1983. Cervical cancer is an insidious chronic disease that can have a long incubation period. Researchers in several countries are working to develop a prototype vaccine, but no such quick fix existed to help me now.

*I didn't know sexual choices made over thirty years ago could affect my reproductive health today.* But what I didn't know could literally kill me.

A surfing expedition on the Internet revealed the terrible death toll. Cervical cancer kills a quarter of a million women each year. In this modern age, the statistics staggered my wildest imagination. Shattered families litter the global landscape as doctors identify half a million new cases annually. Voluminous data from the International Agency for Research on Cancer (IARC) spoke with authority: roughly 80 percent of the new cases (over 400,000 women) occurred in less developed countries each year. Where

Pap tests are widely unavailable, cervical cancer is the number one killer of women worldwide. Women with cervical cancer in these counties have a higher death *rate* than women with breast cancer. What were women doing in Africa, Asia, Central and South America, the Caribbean, and Eastern Europe where the highest incidence and mortality rates occur? *What treatment are they getting,* I wondered aloud? Were they living without hope and dying without Christ? What about the Pap test?

According to data from the National Cancer Institute about 4,100 women die from cervical cancer in the United States, with about 12,200 new cases annually. American physicians attribute the lower incidence to the widespread availability of the Pap test. But my Pap test just 10 months earlier had been completely normal . . . just like the one's I had over the past 25 years. In my case, this routine screening proved useless in early detection and worthless as an indicator of progressive disease. I struggled to understand HPV's latency period and its impact on what I knew was a faithful marriage for the past 26 years. With Amos' help, I learned about the importance of multilayered screening, which combines the Pap test with HPV screening and a diagnostic biopsy. The value of a tiered approach cannot be overstated. But it was too late for that now.

*Lord, Lord Jesus. Please help me get through this!*


Early on Monday before leaving to see the oncologist, Amos led the morning prayers. We both thanked God for His full armor. Armed with information and pertinent questions to clarify confusion regarding the diagnosis, I remembered the Girl Scout motto: be prepared. We waited almost thirty minutes before a nurse called me. She ushered us into a large conference room. It seems there had been yet another mix-up: the oncologist was not in the office, and he wasn't even expected. Instead, his nursing assistant would answer our questions. A new staff member in training joined us as well. Seated in a semicircle, the three of us listened intently as the nursing assistant explained treatment protocols for chemotherapy and radiation. She also advised us of the first oncologist's subsequent referral to another specialist, a radiation oncologist. Taking yet another liberty, she had already scheduled an appointment with this second oncologist on Tuesday, December 26.

*This isn't right, Lord.*

We listened in tacit agreement until she handed me a sheet requiring my signature. Though barely legible, the handwritten entry next to the diagnosis line read: uterine cancer.

*Something's way out of line here, Lord. You are not the author of confusion.*

"The oncologist said I had cervical cancer," I said bluntly. "There's been a mistake." The word "cancer" rolled off my tongue more easily now. It was still heavy, but with repeated usage, it had somehow become much less troublesome and offensive.

"I can't speak for the doctor . . ."

"You seem to be doing a pretty good job," Amos interrupted.

We left the office, convinced I needed to talk with the missing gynecological oncologist as soon as possible. One thing was clear, however, the list of chemotherapy's side effects was enough to curl my hair . . . if I had any hair left once treatments ended.

*Lord, you've given me this hair. Can I please keep it? Thank you!*

Amos and I returned home convinced HUP should be our next stop in the search for a definitive diagnosis. I expected my friend's visit to commence within the next thirty minutes, so I decided to wait until later to place the call. I did leave a message for the gynecological oncologist, however. I needed to know why this first specialist changed his diagnosis from cervical to uterine cancer. It was lunchtime, but once again, I wasn't very hungry.

Before the doorbell rang, I saw my friend's car pull into the driveway. She slammed the door with one hand and carried a cheery poinsettia arrangement in the other. Her bouncy demeanor contrasted sharply with my waning energy. I swung the front door open wide. We greeted one another with warmth and affection. It had been a long time.

"You look terrific," I gushed.

"And you look thin. What's going on?"

Amos and Lorraine formed a welcome committee in the foyer. We all embraced warmly.

"I was just going to get some lunch. Are you hungry?"

"Nope. Let's just use the time to talk," she suggested and immediately made herself at home as she headed to the downstairs family room.

Her ease and grace had a positive, calming effect. We joked about scarlet letters and social stigmas. From a clinical standpoint, she asked if the top or the bottom of the cervix was affected. I didn't have the slightest clue. Reaching into her handbag, she produced three bottles of herbal supplements and two jars of tablets to boost my weakened immune system. She said they would be effective. I gave her my undivided attention.

"Just get as much information as you can and definitely get a second opinion and a third, if necessary. And get some rest. You need to rest," she repeated.

After she left, I called Dr. Zalut's office again. Yes, I needed rest, but not before arranging the electronic referral for the visit with the radiation oncologist and confirming arrangements for the two diagnostic tests. Moving through the late-afternoon hours, I couldn't shake a nagging suspicion. Did the cancer specialists on the New Jersey side of the Walt Whitman Bridge hope to provide treatment without the benefit of a second opinion?

The next step became crystal clear. I called a gynecologist at the Hospital of the University of Pennsylvania (HUP). Five years ago, he and his associates at HUP had taken the most complete health history I had ever experienced. Having lived in California, Illinois, Rhode Island, Washington, D.C., and now New Jersey, I had benefited from treatment at some of the country's major health centers. Today, right now, I needed something more than I'd initially received from the first oncologist.

I left a message for the HUP doctor. In less than thirty minutes, he returned my call. I explained the situation and told him I needed a definitive diagnosis before proceeding. Although he had not seen me in five years, his compassionate words struck a chord.

"I know how hard this is," he began. "We want to help you through this."

He referred me to a physician at HUP whose office returned my call within five minutes. I scheduled an appointment in three days, the coming Thursday. The understanding HUP gynecologist called later in the evening to ensure I'd been contacted. After talking with an associate, he highly recommended a visit to one of the three gynecological oncologists on staff at HUP. Two were males.

The next morning, I called HUP's gynecological oncology department and scheduled an appointment for Wednesday, December

27 with the female specialist. The receptionist instructed me to bring the CT scan films and report, the biopsy slides and report, and the office notes from the gynecological oncologist and the gynecologist who had examined me when the discharge first appeared. Next, I called Dr. Zalut's office again for the required referral. *They're probably getting sick of me asking for all these referrals*, I thought.

With Christmas just six days away, the following week's schedule was filling up as quickly as the week before. And I still had unfinished business on this week's "to do" list. I had not reached the first oncologist, and he had not returned my calls.

*When am I supposed to rest, Lord? Please show me your way to abundant life.*

The schedule for the week ahead at least proved I was alive! Monday was Christmas Day, and on Tuesday, I had an appointment with a radiation oncologist. On Wednesday, I'd meet the gynecological oncologist at HUP. On Thursday, I eagerly anticipated my hairdresser appointment, so I'd look lovely for our twenty-sixth wedding anniversary celebration that evening. On Friday, the girls and I planned a theatrical outing with our church youth group. On Saturday, I looked forward to hosting our holiday party for seven other couples, and Sunday was New Year's Eve.

*Lord Jesus, you know all about this. You have a plan for my life. You know I can only do this if you help me.*

On Thursday, I called Dr. Zalut's referral coordinator to confirm completion of referrals for the next day's CT scan and next week's consultations with the two oncologists. With Christmas on Monday, there was no room for referral error. Everything had to be in place. The referral coordinator confirmed the electronic referrals, and then her next remark floored me.

"You've been approved for visits to the radiation oncologist," she said.

"Visits? What visits?" I asked, nearly speechless from this vicious uppercut to the chin.

She told me the radiation oncologist's office faxed the request on December 15, the day after the first oncologist examined me.

"You've been approved for forty consultations and twenty radiation treatments," she explained. "The visits are good for ninety days," she continued.

"I didn't authorize any visits. I haven't even seen the doctor. When did this happen?" I asked incredulously, struggling to comprehend this knockout punch below the belt.

"This was processed December 18," she said.

*Lord God Almighty, are these people trying to pull a fast one? Will you direct my steps, Lord? I don't even know the diagnosis yet. Don't they know who I am? I'm a child of the King! Help me, Lord. Thank you for helping me.*

I closed the door on BTS Enterprises early Thursday morning, December 21, and attended a prayer luncheon at my friend Lora's home at noon. For the past year, a few women friends gathered periodically for food, fellowship, and fervent prayer. I was the first to arrive, and Lora immediately sent me on an errand to a nearby bakery. When I inadvertently passed the parking lot entrance, I proceeded to the traffic light and flicked the left-turn signal. Waiting for the green arrow, I eagerly anticipated this time of fellowship with Jackie, Lora, and Stephanie, my sisters in Christ from Asbury United Methodist. Lora's cousin Thelma, a hair stylist and salon owner, rounded out the prayer circle. I had already broken the news to Lora over the telephone. Now the others needed to know.

*I'll tell them about the diagnosis, and we'll pray to our heavenly Father,* I thought as I waited for the light to change. The green arrow took an inordinately long time to drop. When I entered the bakery, an elderly couple just couldn't seem to make up their minds between the baklava and the cheesecake. Finally, the patient clerk filled Lora's order for bagels and pastries. I left the fragrant shop carrying a small white box neatly tied with string. At just that moment, an elderly woman approached and headed toward the parking lot with me.

"Hello," she said cheerfully

Smiling, I returned her greeting. "Beautiful day, isn't it?"

The woman struck up a conversation, and I engaged her. She looked forward to celebrating Christmas. Her name was Helen, the same as my mother's. Twelve years ago to the day workmen lowered my mother's casket into the ground. At her funeral service the evening before, my family celebrated mom's life. Touching tributes stirred a standing room only crowd of relatives and friends who came from near and far to honor her memory. Helen McCullough possessed a deep spiritual awareness. Her sense of humor, commitment, and endurance for the heavenly reward were widely recognized. Her faith in Jesus Christ influenced a wide circle and constituted a priceless inheritance. For reasons I cannot explain, I told this stranger I had recently been diagnosed with cancer.

"Oh, I had that, and it went away," she told me.

Back at Lora's house, I rejoiced to tell my friends I believed God heals cancer. I trusted our heavenly Father to take care of me, like He promised. I solicited their prayers with thanksgiving for how God would work things out. We stood holding hands and praying in a circle of love I'll never forget.

That evening, I prepared for the CT scan of the pelvis the next day. Computerized tomography, abbreviated CT, is a radiological imaging test that takes pictures of cross sections of the body. Since scans of the pelvis require an empty lower intestine, I had to drink a barium laxative to clear my colon from top to bottom. I premixed the solution as directed to fill a plastic gallon jug. The instructions required drinking an eight-ounce glass every ten minutes until the entire solution was finished. I never knew ten minutes could pass so quickly. The first few glasses went down easily, but as the rumbling in my intestines increased, I could have saved steps by staying in the bathroom. In the morning, I was weak from fasting as well as the diarrhea. I prepared for the trip to the radiology center, a ten-minute drive from home.

Once inside the room with the scanner, the nursing assistant handed me a white Styrofoam cup.

"You have to drink all of this," she said.

"Not the barium milk shake. Didn't I drink enough last night?" I moaned.

The CT scan required an IV injection of an iodine contrast dye. I sensed the warm flow immediately as the dye entered my veins. Skilled hands manipulated the controls, and I glided inside the doughnut-shaped CT machine. The test took about thirty minutes. I requested a copy of the report and the films in preparation for the next week's appointments with the radiation oncologist and the gynecological oncologist at HUP.

"You might have some stomach discomfort after this is over," the nurse advised me.

*That isn't what the Internet reported,* I thought. I was supposed to resume normal activities without restriction.

*Lord Jesus, I guess I won't be doing too much shopping today, after all.*

Amos strongly suggested we return home instead of shopping. It was lunchtime, and for once, I was actually hungry. He fixed simple fare: soup and a turkey sandwich. I ate with gusto. Over twenty-four hours had passed since my last meal. For a change, we ate in the dining room. Although it was a chilly thirty-five degrees, the afternoon sun shone brightly through elegant French doors. The sound of the doorbell interrupted our impromptu tête-à-tête.

"Who knows we're even home at this hour?" I wondered aloud.

Amos returned with a stunning arrangement of red and white roses in a clear cylindrical vase. Before he could place them on the table, I felt my stomach cramp with merciless urgency. Discomfort jolted my belly like the flash of a lightening bolt.

"Ohhhhh. Those are simply beautiful," I moaned, suddenly woozy. The downward spiral was painful and quick. I could barely lift my head, which rolled from side to side on an outstretched arm. "Who sent them?" I murmured.

The floral spectacle filled the space and the room with an aroma, warmth, and a splash of color that literally took my breath away.

"Amos, I've got to get upstairs. I'm going to be sick. Who knew to send me flowers at just this exact moment?"

*Dear God, you know I love flowers.*

Our friends and former neighbors who now live in Florida sent the colorful arrangement. "Get well soon, love, Jim and Christine," Amos read from the attached card.

"That woman is just so thoughtful. Please help me to the bathroom. I've got to get upstairs."

Our split-level home lacked one critical feature: a first-floor bathroom. I struggled upstairs, leaning heavily on Amos's arm. I had to hurry.

Plagued with yet another bout of diarrhea, I stumbled into the bathroom with no time to spare. Christmas Day was Monday, just three short days away. I had yet to purchase even the first Christmas present.

# Chapter 5

## Second and Third Opinions

⌕ But if he will not hear thee, then take with thee, that in the mouth of two or three witnesses every word may be established.

*Matthew 18:16*

By the grace of God, I survived the barium milk shake cramps. Early Saturday morning, Thom pampered me with a salon manicure and eyebrow wax. Next, I finally went shopping and selected presents for Lorraine, Dana, and Amos. I had no real energy for anything or anyone else. At least there would be something under the tree from me. I also picked up the chest X-ray films and CT scan report from the radiology center. I intuitively felt this was a "good" report. Later that evening, I called my friend who brought the poinsettia. What a blessing to laugh and talk with someone who understood what I was going through.

For the first time in memory, we all slept late Christmas Day and didn't open presents until after eleven o'clock. I experienced the joy of relaxing and getting some really restful sleep on and off all afternoon while the girls prepared dinner. I was more tired than I cared to admit. When I finally ventured downstairs and looked into the dining room, my head spun in quick double-take fashion. With Jim and Christine's red and white roses taking center stage, the elegant china, tapered candles, and folded napkins tied with gold ribbons looked exquisite.

"Ohhhh. How lovely," I exclaimed.

"Merry Christmas," Lorraine and Dana echoed gaily in unison as I entered the kitchen.

"Something smells wonderful," I intoned, relishing the tempting aroma of baked ham and sweet potatoes.

After dinner, my next-door neighbor Marilyn dropped by to wish us Merry Christmas. She stayed for tea and a slice of Lorraine's homemade orange chocolate cake. We enjoyed the festive atmosphere at the dining room table. Without fanfare, Marilyn handed me a neatly wrapped present.

"This is for you."

I tore the colored paper and read the book cover: *Prayers for a Woman of Faith,* a collection of scripture verses. *That's me,* I thought. *Just what I needed.*

"When I saw it, I thought of you immediately," she said.

*Lord, thank you for blessing me with such wonderful friends and neighbors. I pray I never get cocky and take your love for granted. Teach me how to pray as you take me farther on this faith journey. Thank you for going ahead and being with me along every step of the way.*

After Marilyn left, we all trooped downstairs to enjoy the cozy fire and relax. Amos read the Bible's Christmas story from the book of Luke, a family tradition dating back to the days when the girls were toddlers. Next, Dana continued with Matthew's account of Christ's death, and Lorraine read passages concerning the resurrection of Jesus. Then, to my surprise, Lorraine suggested and read from the Revelation of John who wrote about the hope and promise that Christ will come quickly.

In the warm, ambient firelight, the four of us talked for a long while about the goodness of God during the past twelve months. Amos praised God for the completion of his Denver assignment 1,500 miles away and his new job at Lockheed, barely a fifteen-minute drive from home. He also remembered God's grace for the new roof on the house, paid in full. Lorraine thanked God for getting her driver's license, for completing high school, and for the wonderful graduation garden party in June.

We laughed as we remembered her remark that day: "I don't even recognize my own backyard."

Lorraine also praised God for new beginnings and scholarships at Cornell. Dana expressed gratitude for an end to stressful times during the first four months of the year, for the beginning of voice lessons with Lin Krupa, and for the transition into her new role as "only child."

I listened with joy and didn't have too much more to add when my turn rolled around. They had said it all. Sure, BTS enjoyed another good year. We were still in business, praise the Lord. If I had a thousand tongues, I couldn't thank our clients enough for their continuing support and trust. I had attended a writer's conference in July but still had not developed the discipline, motivation, or diligence to sustain a serious writing project. But mostly, I simply affirmed love for my family through it all. We were not just four people at a bus stop. Inextricably linked, yet distinctly individual, each member of the family gave shape and texture to a complex network of relationships. The whole really is greater than the sum of the parts. Unraveling the roles of husband and wife, father and daughter(s), mother and daughter(s), sisters, and *self* was enough to drive me batty sometimes. Thank God I didn't drink! Sometimes I wondered aloud if I was in the "right" family, but tonight I knew I was. Surely, God had provided the right people for the job.

*Help us, Holy Ghost, to make sense of the past, and then forget it. Help us to look forward with enthusiasm to the new thing you are doing in our midst.*

Impatient for conversation to end, Dana flipped the remote control to start an annual tradition. It was time to enjoy the feature film: *It's a Wonderful Life.*

The next morning, Amos and I prepared for the ten o'clock appointment with the radiation oncologist. I still had not reached the first gynecological oncologist despite repeated calls. We arrived at the specialist's office about fifteen minutes before the scheduled appointment. Although the receptionist seemed somewhat agitated, the friendly folks in the waiting room exuded warmth and enthusiasm.

"So how was your holiday?" I asked no one in particular.

A middle-aged woman with a kind smile talked about the delicious Christmas dinner and decorations at her daughter-in-law's house. A portly man with a cane laughed about board games he played with his grandchildren. They each seemed to know one another, greeting newcomers by name as they entered. With a schedule of daily radiation treatments, it was only natural to become acquainted with those who were treated at the same time, I surmised. I completed the blanks on the patient questionnaire. When the nursing assistant called me, I entered the maze of inner offices. She ushered Amos and me into a conference room, and we awaited the familiar knock. I asked Amos if he cared to observe the pelvic exam. He was noncommittal.

In his early forties, the oncologist radiated cordiality as he extended his hand in greeting.

"So how are you today?" he asked with a smile.

"I showed up, Doc," I answered cheerfully.

"So what's been happening?" he asked.

I recounted the details with specificity and professionalism. The doctor listened intently as I explained the confusion in the diagnosis. Although I had tried repeatedly to reach the first oncologist by phone for over a week, he had not yet returned my calls. This new specialist discussed the different treatment protocols for cervical versus endometrial or uterine cancer. Cervical cancer is typically treated with chemotherapy and both external and internal radiation to the pelvis, he said. Uterine cancer most often requires a total hysterectomy followed by radiation treatments, if there is spread to the lymph nodes, he explained.

The doctor surmised I had uterine cancer on the basis of the biopsy and the CT scan. But he cautiously reserved final judgment until he conducted a pelvic exam supported by results of magnetic resonance imaging or MRI of the pelvis. The MRI would provide more detailed soft-tissue analysis than what is usually observed on the CT scan, he said. He wrote a prescription for the MRI on the spot. In the next breath, the specialist apologized for the absence of his regular nurse who was out sick for the day. He needed to examine me and would find a stand-in staffer.

Amos expressed reservations about the pelvic exam. "She's going to be seen at HUP tomorrow and will most likely be treated there," he said. "You're not a gynecologist," my husband added.

I understood instinctively. My dear husband didn't want this strange man looking at private, intimate parts typically reserved for his eyes only. The oncologist expressed concern for his professional reputation.

If I showed up at the hospital where he received his training, and he had failed to examine me, "I'd be a laughing stock," he said.

*Lord, will you help these two men put their personal interests on the back burner for a minute. There are complicated relationships all around, Father.*

"Look . . . I just want to clarify this confusion," I interjected. "Let's just get the diagnosis right, so I can move on."

This was what was at stake for me, and I wasn't afraid to say so: I had already undergone one C-section in 1982. There was another C-section in 1985, which included tubal ligation and a third surgery only three days after delivering Dana when the abdominal incision ruptured. Those were some difficult, painful days. I didn't get the bikini cut. With a low pain threshold to boot, I was wary of tearing open old scars. With a diagnosis of cervical cancer, another abdominal surgery would not be necessary, if I understood the options correctly. Chemotherapy and radiation treatments would do the job. If, on the other hand, the diagnosis was uterine cancer, and surgery was unavoidable, then so be it. I'd start chemotherapy after that. Whatever clinical examinations and diagnostic tests were necessary to reach the best professional diagnosis and individualized treatment protocol, then bring it on. "Next" typified my attitude in business and household matters, and this was no different.

"Do you mind giving us a few moments alone?" I asked politely.

The doctor approached the door and apologized again for his nurse's absence. "I'll just set up the exam room and warm the speculum," he said flatly before closing the door.

"I'm not comfortable with this exam," Amos confided.

I took a deep breath. His comfort was the least of my concerns at that moment. *His* feet weren't going in the stirrups.

"Look, Amos. This exam is important. It's part of the deal. I need to be examined again so this doc can make a determination," I stated firmly. "When I told this man I had 'shown up,' that's what I meant. I understand I'm not necessarily going to be comfortable. But I am going to carry on with the next step, and this is it," I exhaled, holding nothing back.

"Are you going to come in?" I asked in the heavy silence.

"I'm going," Amos agreed, opening the door. I detected no trace of reluctance.

*Thank you, Lord.*

The radiation oncologist reentered the conference room and led the way to a small exam room. He handed me a gown.

After a few minutes, he returned with a female radiation therapist he had drafted to assist with the pelvic exam. Wearing a white lab coat and a cheerful smile, she shook my extended hand. Right away, Amos noticed the bounty of colored markers clipped to her lab coat pocket. Amos, eccentric engineer that he is, has a penchant for assorted pens, pencils, and markers. He immediately started a conversation with the therapist about her collection. The doctor adjusted my feet in the stirrups.

"I use these pens to mark a patient's body," she explained. On the Internet, I learned about technicians who used tiny dots of colored, semipermanent ink to outline the treatment area. These tattoos indicate the exact place on a patient's body where machines aim high-powered rays.

*Amos needs a distraction, Lord. Help him, Holy Ghost. Heaven help us all.*

With rapt attention, Amos continued his line of questioning like a reporter on deadline. At this point, my own curiosity surfaced and pulled me into the act.

"Are they permanent markers that will eventually wear off?" I asked.

"No, I mark with these and then we apply a permanent tattoo," she explained.

The oncologist finished positioning me on the table. Ready to start, he closed the door on further conversation.

"If you like, we'll tattoo Amos," he suggested.

"I really don't think that will be necessary," I said dryly.

When the laughter subsided, Amos moved into position behind the doctor's right shoulder. The curtain rose on this opening scene and the show began. The doctor spread the labia with gloved fingers and inserted a warm speculum into the vagina. The sympathetic soul with the pens moved closer and held my hand.

"Are you all right?" she asked sincerely.

"Even though I'm almost fifty years old and have two children," I replied, "I'll never be comfortable with this exam." She nodded knowingly.

The radiation oncologist carefully explained every step of the examination. Using a light to illuminate the vaginal walls, he turned briefly to Amos and said, "Now here's the cervix and . . ."

"It looks pretty healthy to me," Amos interrupted triumphantly.

For the first time in my life, I laughed out loud during a pelvic exam . . . a deep belly laugh that broke all tension. Amos's remark caught the medical professionals completely off guard. They laughed too.

*Unforgettable, Lord. That's my man. My "MOS man!"*

The doctor resumed his professional demeanor. He agreed that, indeed, the cervical tissue did look normal . . . pink with no lesions. Removing the speculum, he inserted the index and middle fingers into the vagina and pressed firmly on my abdomen to feel for any abnormalities of the uterus or ovaries. Then he examined the rectum. *At least he didn't have a three-finger trick up his sleeve*, I thought with gratitude. Finished, he removed the rubber gloves with a snap.

"You can get dressed now. I'll be back."

*Thank you, Jesus. That's over.*

When the doctor returned, he told us he felt no perimetrial extension on the left side. He could not feel anything to confirm the first oncologist's diagnosis. He held the CT scan films up to the light. This specialist repeated that an MRI should definitely be done to confirm the diagnosis.

"Are you married, Doctor?" I asked.

Extending his left hand, the oncologist explained how he stopped wearing his wedding ring because he had recently undergone surgical removal of a bump on his finger.

"Okaaaay," I said slowly with a puzzled look on my face. I had not bargained for all that. "I just wanted to know, if your wife presented with this, where would you recommend that she be treated? Which hospital?"

"Penn," he said without a moment's hesitation.

Later that evening, Lora telephoned, and we talked about the prophet Jonah. He wanted to run away and not hear God's message or give it to others, but God had another plan for him. We also talked about the joy of the friendship we shared. We both praised the Lord Jesus for being the only God with power to take us beyond the brink when life had us on the edge. After our conversation, I reflected on what I faced. *Forget any lack of clarity on the diagnosis,* I thought. I needed a clear picture of *myself* . . . of all God had done in me and through me over the years to prepare me for the days ahead . . . to prepare for tomorrow's visit to yet another oncologist and another pelvic exam for heaven's sake.

*If the joy of the Lord is my strength, then I'd better get prepared to be deliriously joyful. I needed strength,* I thought with a sigh. Anything that looked or even smelled like fear had to move out of the way.

*I tell you the truth, if you have faith as small as a mustard seed, you can say to this mountain, "Move from here to there," and it will move. Nothing will be impossible for you.*

Something a dear friend wrote about me in 1997 came to mind. Fishing through a bureau drawer to find it, I reread her words with a grateful heart.

*She fills me with joy and my heart is overflowing, in her words everything is new. Hope is abounding. Life is a work in progress to be inhaled, exhaled, experienced (no too calm a word). Absorbed through every pore. In her words the Lord is alive and the possibilities endless. Bigger, and so much bigger than I had ever imagined. Taken to a high place, encouraged, and set free. Irene!*

*Yes, that's who I am!* I refolded her note. I thanked God for family and friends who loved me. *Jesus loves me, this I know.* So I could definitely love myself.

Bright and early the next day, Amos and I listened to the morning news and dressed for the trip to Philadelphia. I wore an olive pantsuit with a herringbone pattern. Taking time and effort to look stylish encouraged me. Because appearance also affects the perception of others, I hoped to look and sound coherent for this first meeting with the second gynecological oncologist.

After parking in Penn Towers, we walked across "The Bridge," a glass-enclosed overhead walkway spanning Spruce Street that connected the parking garage and medical offices to the hospital. The bridge afforded shelter, particularly on cold, windy days like today. We entered the hospital and headed toward the doctor's office. With several interconnected buildings, the Hospital of the University of Philadelphia is a winding maze of corridors and offices. The marble floors on the remodeled second floor shine like glass. I'd find this specialist in the Courtyard Building, not far from the information desk near the bridge entrance. The receptionist greeted us warmly. Her name was Dana.

"That's easy to remember. My daughter's name is Dana," I said.

I handed her the large envelope containing the CT scan films, the biopsy slides, related reports, and two sets of office notes, one from the first gynecological oncologist and another from the gynecologist who examined me following the initial discharge in November. Dana handed me the all-too-familiar patient questionnaire. I took a seat and discretely observed the women in the waiting room, especially those with their husbands or significant others.

*I don't guess anyone is here unless they have to be, Lord.*

When the nurse announced my name, I stood with Amos, and she ushered us into a small consultation room. We waited almost thirty minutes before the doctor tapped politely and entered with my paperwork in hand. After making introductions, she apologized for the delay caused by an emergency. Small framed with delicate features and Caribbean Sea blue eyes, she looked to be in her mid to late thirties. Trained in gynecologic oncology at Johns Hopkins School of Medicine, she was an assistant professor at the University of Pennsylvania School of Medicine. Settling comfortably behind the desk, she leaned forward.

"What's been going on?" she asked.

By this time, I felt like I was reading from a script. Sounding like a broken record, I recounted the specific details from the onset of the discharge to yesterday's visit with the radiation oncologist. The doctor sketched a crude diagram of the reproductive anatomy on a pharmaceutical notepad. She explained my options, in much the same way as the first gynecological oncologist and the radiation oncologist had done. Before she could make a definitive diagnosis, however, she needed to examine me.

*Here we go again, Lord.*

Though I was modestly draped, once the sheet was turned back, I simply lay naked and spread-eagle exposed for yet another doctor to see and touch. While the specialist showed compassion, that didn't diminish her professional obligation to probe aggressively for the existence and spread of an insidious and deadly disease.

"Has anyone ever mentioned you have fibroids?" she asked.

"Fibroids? No, no one ever said anything about fibroids," I stammered, struggling to maintain composure on the exam table once again.

Well no . . . no one had *ever* mentioned fibroids. I had monitored my reproductive health as regularly as I knew how. Yet, here she was telling me of yet another problem that had escaped detection despite four recent pelvic examinations conducted by three different doctors.

*I'm not feeling this, Lord.*

"Is it ever customary for a gynecologist to insert fingers in the rectum and vagina at the same time during an exam?" I asked when she finished and I was sitting upright. I could change the subject with the best of them.

"Sometimes it is done. Why?"

"That's what happened with the first oncologist who examined me," I explained. *He certainly didn't say anything about any fibroids,* I thought with distaste.

"Why don't you get dressed, and we'll talk more," she said simply.

*Is this what they teach them in medical school, Father?*

I rejoined Amos who was waiting in the consultation room. About ten minutes later, the oncologist continued the consultation. She was virtually certain I had uterine cancer and needed a total hysterectomy.

"I can do the surgery on Friday, the day after tomorrow," she offered.

*What is this, Lord? A year-end clearance special?*

"Whoa, there," I responded. "That's just a little too soon," I added. We had plans for our wedding anniversary the next day and theater plans with our church youth group on Friday. The doctor appeared disinterested. For heaven's sake, our holiday party was scheduled for Saturday evening. I wasn't canceling the plans. Uterine cancer or cervical cancer or whatever I had didn't exactly fit my schedule at the moment. Besides, I needed time to pray and think and do some research.

"Do you recommend an MRI?" I asked.

"No, you don't really need one. We have our weekly conference on Friday, and I'll bring your case up then. I'm also going to have another pathologist look at the biopsy slides," she explained.

"The radiation oncologist told me yesterday an MRI would definitively confirm the diagnosis," I said. "How can you be sure?"

"No, I don't think the MRI is really necessary because the pathology report indicates there is cancer in the uterus. That's not in question. You will need a hysterectomy, but the actual grading of disease and sampling of the lymph nodes will take place when the surgery is performed."

Amos, visibly uncomfortable, had some questions. The specialist discussed cure rates and survival percentages, but her numbers and calculations went completely over my head. This *one* just wanted to live.

On the drive back home, Amos and I spoke very little. The towering spans of the Walt Whitman Bridge stood stark against a brilliant blue sky.

"You know, when I talked to Susan, I told her I didn't want to start any treatments until the holidays were over and everyone had sobered up," I said offhandedly. "Guess what she said? 'You got that right. And before they get their Visa bill, you have to time this thing right,'" I added. "Look, our anniversary is tomorrow. Friday, the girls and I will be gone all day, and the party is Saturday. Let's just praise God for one day at a time and enjoy it," I suggested.

With one hand firmly on the wheel, Amos flicked the steering column switch to increase the volume on the radio. Changing lanes to pass a slow driver, we entered New Jersey and prepared for the last four days before the new millennium. At this juncture in the road, three oncologists had examined me, but no two had reached the same conclusion. The first one diagnosed cervical cancer and wanted to begin chemotherapy and radiation treatments the next week. Unfortunately, nine days had passed without a single returned phone call. The second specialist could not confirm either cervical or uterine cancer. He reserved judgment until he could examine the MRI test results. Now, a third oncologist had diagnosed uterine cancer, discovered fibroids, and wanted to perform a hysterectomy at the drop of a hat.

*What am I supposed to make of all this, Lord?*

The first oncologist never even mentioned an MRI, and the third one didn't even think an MRI was necessary. The first oncologist, who examined me two weeks ago, puzzled me the most. *Why hadn't he returned my calls,* I wondered. *I'll try again tomorrow,* I thought, as we got closer to home. Tomorrow is my twenty-sixth wedding anniversary.

Amos and I planned to hear a popular jazz saxophonist to celebrate our anniversary. After twenty-six years of marriage, I not only loved Amos, I *still* liked him. Through the thick and the thin, and certainly in sickness and in health, God kept us together. I intended to celebrate God's faithfulness. This was *His* marriage, after all. He joined us together, and for better or worse, richer or poorer, we had managed to find something to laugh about for over a quarter of a century. My hairdresser expected me at the salon at eleven o'clock, and I didn't want to be late. My hair needed primping to look especially flattering for the evening ahead. I wanted to feel relaxed, joyful, *and* beautiful. It was a tall order on the heels of all that had occurred in recent days, but I believe Jesus and a hot curling iron in the hands of a skilled professional can work wonders to provide peace and contentment through life's trials.

Only a few clients patronized La Pearl's Beauty Emporium that Thursday morning. Sitting in the salon chair, Pearl and I chatted easily about our respective Christmas celebrations with our families. She gently brushed through medium-length black hair with one hand and waved the blow dryer nozzle back and forth with the other. On the last salon visit, when I told her about the cancer diagnosis, she showed compassion by graciously offering to go wig shopping with me *before* I needed one.

Suddenly, the unexpected thrust of an intensely sharp pain on the left side of my chest interrupted any thought of wigs or anniversary plans. Wincing, I clutched my chest with my right hand under the protective black vinyl cape and pressed hard. Just as suddenly, pinpricks jabbed my left hand, and a steady numbing stream moved rapidly up the left arm.

*What's happening, Lord? There's just never a dull moment, I tell you! I cannot have a heart attack now!*

*I gotta get my hair done. I'm going out tonight*, I thought frantically. Then, as surreptitiously as possible, I repeatedly flexed my hand and pumped my arm as discreetly as I could under the cape. All the while, I fervently prayed for the heavenly Father's help with every squeeze. *No panicking! I will not panic, Lord. I'm going out tonight! Please help me!*

Absently stroking the dryer nozzle through my hair, Pearl seemed oblivious to my painful dilemma. *I have to drive back home*, I thought, privately pumping my arm. I know God heard those prayers because I eased from the chair, collected belongings, and drove home from West Philadelphia to New Jersey without incident. At least my hair looked great. To return safely across the bridge proved God's grace yet again. When I reached the house, the chest pain subsided, but the numbness and tingling continued. Then, to my utter amazement, my hand turned blue and literally shriveled up before my eyes.

*Lord Jesus. You helped the man with the withered hand. You healed him! So I know you can take care of mine.*

I called Dr. Zalut, my primary care physician. I wasn't going to anybody's emergency room. I had no intention of spending four or five hours in ER on my anniversary. Unfortunately, I couldn't get through to the doctor. Instead, I worked that left hand with one of those stress balls all afternoon and hoped the doctor would call me back. When the telephone rang and Dana announced it was the doctor, I didn't expect the first oncologist to identify himself.

"I've tried to reach you repeatedly," I began.

"I sent you a fax," he said.

"I didn't receive it, Doctor. Please hold on."

I called for Dana to check the fax machine in the office. She returned with a two-page letter addressed to Dr. Stanley, my gynecologist. I quickly perused the contents. Dated December 26 and faxed on December 27, the letter read in part: "It is my impression that probably Irene has stage IIB adenocarcinoma of the uterus."

*The uterus?*

The first oncologist had flip-flopped on this original diagnosis. The Spirit, the precious and powerful Holy Spirit, gave me the right words to say during our brief conversation.

*Thank you, Lord Jesus, for allowing me to speak to him. You taught me how to do that, and you used a loving mother who insisted her daughters speak graciously.*

I rested after lunch, and then dressed for our special date. I tried again to reach Dr. Zalut, without success. We left home around six o'clock and stopped at his office en route to Philadelphia.

"He's with a patient and can't see you now," the receptionist politely informed me.

Squeezing the stress ball and laughing my head off, I crossed the Walt Whitman Bridge for the third time in one day and enjoyed a wonderful evening with the man I love! I had so much fun despite the numbness, the bone-chilling temperatures, and the blustery wind gusts. This was our first excursion to this heavily advertised theater. I praised God I decided not to wear a dressy coat because the place was so raunchy. In characteristic fashion, Amos joked that it would be a miracle if we got out of the building before it was condemned! I worked the stress ball during the entire performance, thoroughly enjoying every minute of Amos's joviality, as much as the first half of the show. At intermission, a long line of women waited to enter the ladies' room.

"This is disgusting," I said to no one in particular. I sidestepped puddles of water on the floor and gave a sidelong glance at the filthy facilities. There was no point in hesitating . . . I had to go. *I could catch a disease in here*, I mused. Thank God for the tissue in my purse.

The powerhouse jazz sound of the tenor and alto saxophone was enough to blow the roof off the dilapidated theater. The show ended before midnight. The crowd of patrons emptied slowly into the frigid night air. We decided to cross the bridge and get a midnight snack on the New Jersey side, but all the area restaurants closed early. Undaunted, Amos stopped at a local grocery store for peel and eat shrimp and cheesecake. We dined by candlelight on fine china and raised champagne glasses in toast. *Praise God from whom all blessings flow!* The memory of a fun-filled evening at a truly raunchy theater and the lingering melodies of the jazz saxophone would not soon fade.

The next morning, I relished the chance to sleep late. In a few hours, the girls and I would depart with our church youth group to see *The Miracle at Christmas*, a production of the nationally renowned Sight and Sound Theater in Lancaster, Pennsylvania. Lying in bed, I visualized highlights from last night's performance. I felt happy admiring the diamond ring Amos gave me. In March, on the occasion of Lorraine's eighteenth birthday, he replaced the simple gold band I'd worn for 25 years. When the telephone rang, one of the girls answered.

"It's the doctor for you, Mom."

Expecting my primary care physician, I immediately launched into a description of the numbness in my hand. To my surprise, the radiation oncologist who examined me on December 26 identified himself.

"Please forgive me for the confusion. So much has been happening," I apologized.

"I was just calling to see if you're doing okay. Are you getting treatment?" he inquired.

"Thank you for your concern, Doc. Yes, I went to HUP the day after I saw you," I said. "After the New Year, I will probably be treated at HUP. I still want to get an MRI, though," I added.

"Good. That's good. I was just checking some of my files, and I wanted to follow up on you," he said.

I appreciated his concern and informed him the first oncologist who examined me December 14 had changed his diagnosis from cervical to uterine cancer.

"What! I don't believe it. That's incredible," he exclaimed expressing genuine surprise. And then he admitted the fuller extent of his relationship and reliance on the first oncologist for referrals.

"I need him to eat," he said.

*What? Did you hear that, Lord? I don't believe he said that! What do I look like . . . some kind of meal ticket? Help me with this, Father. Please help me.*

When our conversation ended, I clicked off the cordless phone, threw it down on the bed, and shook my head in exasperation.

*Father God. Hear my prayer. I need you, Lord. Will you protect me, Father?*

While it was unclear *why* the first oncologist changed the diagnosis, one thing was certain: I needed God's wisdom to sort out the facts. First, one oncologist didn't bother to return urgent calls for nearly two weeks, then did a complete turnaround on the diagnosis. Then, another oncologist evidently kept a very keen eye on the bottom line. Was I being auctioned to the first lucky bidder for my health care dollars? Was this a case where the early bird treated the cancer worm?

Although there is some disagreement among medical professionals, in many cases, if a biopsy shows uterine cancer, then the standard treatment calls for a hysterectomy followed by chemotherapy and/or radiation. If, on the other hand, doctors uncover cervical cancer, then chemotherapy and radiation are considered the standard of care. Thousands of dollars were on the line . . . cash for Visa payments, new cars, college tuition, stocks and bonds, vacations in Hawaii, and grocery bills. I wasn't begrudging anyone earning a livelihood, but not at the expense of an incorrect diagnosis.

*Help me, Holy Ghost!*

In the next instant, God's Word infiltrated my thinking: *If anyone lacks wisdom let him ask of God who gives liberally . . . but ask in faith or you will get nothing.* Now this was a key I could use. The plain English paraphrase made the point even more succinctly: *If you want to know what God wants you to do, ask him . . .* now that works for me.

Later that Friday afternoon, the girls and I joined our church youth group for the bus trip to Pennsylvania Dutch Country. *The Miracle at Christmas* gives an epic depiction of the Christmas story from the Bible's opening scene in the Garden of Eden, when the Seed was first promised, to the triumphant reign of Christ. When the performance ended, tears of joy streamed down my face. I could not stop crying.

*OUR LORD REIGNS! HE REIGNS!*

In stark contrast to the shabby, neglected building I'd visited the night before, the Sight and Sound Theater stood in a class by itself for excellence. The sets, the sound and lighting effects, and the panoramic stage bombarded the senses. I absorbed the awesome pageantry like a child filled with wonder. There were galloping horses, flying angels, blazing buildings, soaring doves, defeated demons, triumphant believers, and the risen, reigning Christ . . . what a spectacle!

By Saturday, I relished sleeping late again before continuing my steamroller countdown to the New Year. I put finishing touches on the house decorations for our holiday party at seven o'clock and set a gala buffet table for seven couples. But God was in control, not me. Between jazz sets, various radio announcers broadcast cancellations throughout the region. Forecasters expected a major snowstorm to blanket Southern New Jersey and Southeastern Pennsylvania with six to eight inches of powdery flakes.

"Are you canceling the party, Mom?" Dana asked around 4:30 as feathery snowflakes piled higher in the driveway.

"No, I'm having it. Whoever shows up, that's who'll be here," I affirmed.

By 5:30, everyone had called to express regrets. No one dared to venture out in this weather. I lit every candle in the house. A cozy fire blazed brightly. When we clasped hands and thanked the Lord for the food, even Dana thanked God for everyone *He* intended to gather around our table. We feasted, talked, and laughed together. Later that evening I called a trusted friend who encouraged me to consider alternative treatments after the New Year. Around ten o'clock, the numbness in my hand returned, only this time a wave of nausea washed over me. Fighting gravity, yet feeling its unrelenting pull, I grabbed the sides of the chair to keep from fainting.

Amos drove me to the closest hospital emergency room, ten minutes away. Praise God for the triage nurse who determined my condition was urgent. Without much delay, an orderly whisked me away for an EKG. After extensive blood work, a CT scan of the brain, and a chest X-ray, we left the hospital at two o'clock in the morning. To top it all off, my monthly period started . . . of all the crazy, ill-timed things. All tests proved normal, except a precipitously low hemoglobin level, an indication of iron-starved blood and anemia. On the way home from the hospital, Amos said we would not be going to worship service in the morning. No problem . . . I was exhausted.

Early Sunday morning, Amos and I awoke to an insistent knock on our front door. *Who could it possibly be so early*, I wondered? An enterprising man with a snowblower and a boy with a shovel offered to clear the driveway and the front of our house for $20.

Now that the way was cleared, we decided to attend the New Year's Eve morning worship service, after all. Shouts and praises resounded at Asbury that day. Several people gave personal testimonies of the great things God had done during the past year. Together, we committed ourselves to walk by faith in 2001, with the full assurance that what God promised He is able to do!

# Chapter 6

## The Surgery

⸻ Lo, children are a heritage of the Lord: and the fruit of
the womb is his reward.

*Psalm 127:3*

**M**y daughters protested New Year's Eve morning. They were
just too sleepy to attend Sunday worship service with us. Somehow,
they miraculously revived in the afternoon and happily prepared
for sleepover parties. Lorraine planned to spend the evening with
several old high school friends.

"I live in a coed dorm, Mom," Lorraine responded emphatically
when I raised an eyebrow and questioned the sleeping
arrangements. I trusted God for my daughter's integrity. I also knew
the character of some of these young men and women since grade
school. If I couldn't trust Lorraine's judgment at home, then there
was no hope for me while she was away at Cornell.

"It's just girls at my friend's house," Dana assured me quickly
as we discussed her evening plans.

"Thank God," I responded in earnest. I fully trusted God's plan
for Dana too. Both daughters generally exercised good judgment
and I was grateful for their choice of neighborhood friends.

Amos and I enjoyed the holiday at home beside the flickering
amber glow of the fireplace. A calming quietness filled each room.
We read and discussed Psalm 139, then prayed together. Raising

champagne glasses filled to the brim with sparkling cider, we happily toasted the New Year.

"To God's glory and to continuing good health," Amos proposed.

One week ago on Christmas Day, the four of us had looked back on the year with appreciation. Tonight, just the two of us looked ahead with hope in God's mercy for all we could see on the horizon and for what lay hidden beneath the surface. Especially grateful for the growth and maturity of our daughters, we called it a night about half past ten.

On January 2, Amos and I crossed the familiar bridge into Philadelphia. I respected a friend's recommendation to consult an alternative health care professional. Amos remained skeptical but still agreed to accompany me to the midmorning appointment. Shortly after returning home, Amos grabbed a quick lunch, then left for work. I filled the bathtub with steamy hot water and lit a scented candle. There was no good reason not to take full advantage of a quiet bubble bath while the girls were still out shopping. I needed privacy and relaxation to digest all that had transpired since November. I mustered the remnant of scant reserves. "Watch your oil," my mom had often advised. While my supply of proverbial "oil" hovered dangerously close to "empty," I could not and would not put my faith in man . . . any man or any woman.

"I BELIEVE GOD!" I shouted with a loud, strong voice. "I believe GOD."

During the past two weeks, God had spoken to my heart and soul of nothing but healing and comfort. Speaking through his Word the Bible, He provided one key to survival after another. He gave Malachi 4:2: *But unto you that fear my name shall the Sun of righteousness arise with healing in his wings; and ye shall go forth, and grow up as calves of the stall.*

I didn't pretend to understand the part about the calves, but I still received the healing. He offered me *all* of Psalm 91: *He that dwells in the secret place of the most High shall abide under the shadow of the Almighty . . . He is my refuge and my fortress . . .*

I recalled the day, December 14, when Dr. Stanley delivered the news and the first oncologist examined me. On that day, before I even left home, God granted the absolute assurance of Isaiah

43:1-2: . . . *Fear not . . . I have called thee by name; thou art mine. When thou pass through the waters, I will be with thee; and through the rivers, they shall not overflow thee: when thou walk through the fire, neither shall the flame kindle upon thee.*

That settled it. I had God's Word I wouldn't get burned. Several praying friends confirmed God's message.

The warm tub soothed and quieted. Suddenly, I realized that during the past two weeks, while going virtually nonstop, I possessed peace in abundance. The Holy Spirit not only met my need, He provided enough for me to share with many others who needed comfort. As a direct result of breaking the silence about my diagnosis, someone unburdened a load he had shouldered alone for fourteen years! That had to be the grace of God! Not everyone received the news of the cancer diagnosis very well. Some found it just too bitter a pill to hear about, let alone swallow. The hollow sound of some voices spoke volumes. The distant look in certain eyes told a sad tale. Nonetheless, many family members and friends remained open, honest, and supportive during this phase. Their love definitely lifted me. *Love lifts us all!* I thought.

After bathing, I snuggled under warm covers for a late-afternoon nap. Nearly three weeks had transpired since the gynecologist first broke the awful news. Today, I had some news of my own.

"I'm recovering from the *diagnosis* of cancer," I said aloud. "Starting today, I am in recovery." Happy New Year!

The conclusion to what is always a busy and hectic holiday season is Amos's birthday on January 5. I hoped he would enjoy the pageantry and spectacle of the season finale of *Miracle at Christmas* as much as I had the first time.

"Didn't we just go out last week?" he asked as he sped up the highway Saturday evening. "This could become habit forming."

Now that Christmas, my anniversary, New Year's Day, and Amos's birthday celebration were past, it was time to focus on the next faithful steps toward health and wholeness.

First thing Monday morning, I called the same radiology center where I underwent the CT scan to schedule an MRI of the pelvis. While the oncologist at HUP didn't think it was necessary, the radiation oncologist had written the prescription for the procedure back on December 26. I had an ace up my sleeve for this additional diagnostic test, and I planned to use it. The first available opening was January 17. Not as soon as I would have hoped, but I was grateful. Soon afterward, I visited Dr. Zalut about the numbness in my hand and arm.

"You've got a pinched nerve in your elbow," the doctor pronounced. Dr. Zalut expressed much more concern about the anemia. My iron level needed a considerable boost before surgery, or else I might require a blood transfusion, he warned. Early Tuesday morning, I received a call from the surgeon's office to schedule the hysterectomy at HUP. The first available opening was Tuesday, January 23. I immediately correlated this date with Psalm 23: *The Lord is my Shepherd, I shall not want.*

*I shall guide thee continually, Irene.*

I hoped the MRI would miraculously show the tumor had disappeared. Like the three Hebrew boys on the threshold of the fiery furnace, I had a key. I knew God could deliver me from the scalpel, but whether He did or not, I had made up my mind to praise God whatever the outcome. I shared my resolve with a dear friend from upstate New York who remarked that I had "crazy faith."

"Hallelujah anyhow," I said.

As usual, the calendar filled up quickly in the first weeks of January. Out in Chicago, my dad would undergo a minor outpatient surgery on January 17, the same day as my scheduled MRI. Lorraine returned to Cornell on Saturday, January 20. Big sister Sue was slated for foot surgery on Friday, January 26, in Denver. God willing, we planned to celebrate Dana's milestone "sweet sixteen" birthday on Monday, January 29.

In the meantime, the tiredness I experienced as the Christmas season approached paled in comparison to the intense fatigue I now experienced. Anemia and the stress of the unknown wore me down with a vengeance. With my energy level at an all-time low, it was decidedly unwise to forego an afternoon nap. Even around the house, I ordered my steps carefully. Unnecessary trips up and down the stairs were out of the question. God showed mercy because I didn't work outside the home.

I continually affirmed my commitment to praise the Lord when the MRI results were in, whatever they showed. *God calls things that are not as though they were,* I reminded myself constantly. The Lord Jesus is the Creator and great change agent. With four doctors now involved in my care, God sent a fifth gynecologist, Dr. Lyra Gillette, who lived in Los Angeles.

Dr. Gillette is a personal friend of Charlotte's, a dear friend whom Amos and I have known for over twenty years. Our friendship dates back to the days when we lived in San Diego. On January 7, Charlotte called from Los Angeles and talked to Amos for over an hour. Then, I picked up the phone, and she encouraged me to call Dr. Gillette. Somewhat hesitant to introduce yet another professional opinion into the mix, especially across so many miles, I dialed her home number and explained the situation to date. With compassion, understanding, and professionalism, the doctor agreed things were very confused given the original change in the diagnosis. She asked if I'd had a colposcopy, a diagnostic test which uses a colposcope, a lighted microscope, to observe abnormal areas of the vagina and cervix in significantly greater detail. I had never even heard of this test.

In the absence of a colposcopy, Dr. Gillette advised the MRI would be a very important component in reaching an accurate diagnosis by delineating any cervical lesions. She also expressed surprise no one had ever detected fibroids before December 27.

"Do you weigh more than two hundred pounds?" she asked in her lilting Trinidadian accent. Bewildered, I told her I stood five feet seven inches, and weighed a trim 130 pounds.

"Why do you ask?" I said.

"A woman who is overweight or obese is at a much greater risk for these fibroids and also for breast cancer because estrogen is stored in the fat cells," she explained. "This cervical cancer usually presents in third-world countries where women don't have access to a Pap smear. When was your last Pap test?" Dr. Gillette asked.

"I was tested back in January 2000 . . . a year ago . . . and then on December 27," I responded. I had not received a Pap test in November when I first presented with the vaginal discharge. The insurance company would only pay for one test within each twelve-month period.

On Wednesday, January 17, Amos and I headed to the radiology center for the scheduled MRI. Magnetic resonance imaging uses state-of-the-art technology to provide detailed pictures of the internal organs. In my case, the test would depict any cervical lesions or masses within the abdominal cavity.

The immense machinery looked intimidating. A kind nurse offered protective headphones and yet another barium drink. Flat on my back, I glided smoothly into a narrow, hollow tunnel. A sound like hydraulic jackhammers pounded incessantly at periodic intervals. There was no telling what this diagnostic test would reveal. Throughout the procedure, as steady as the hammering cadence, I affirmed my God's ability to save me from the surgical knife and heal the reproductive system He created. But even if He didn't, I was still going to praise Him. *A mighty fortress is our God, a bulwark never failing*, I sang between intervals as the pounding subsided. *Great is thy faithfulness . . . morning by morning new mercies I see*, I sang in the Spirit as the jackhammers pounded. With my mind made up, I trusted this Lord to lead and guide me. I walked by faith and not by sight.

When Saturday, January 20, rolled around, I still had an agenda. I wanted to drive to Ithaca with Amos when he took Lorraine back to school. I hoped to meet the woman with the door key under the jug where we stayed during Cornell's Parent's Weekend. After our bed-and-breakfast stay back in November, I wrote a brief note of appreciation for her hospitality. I also made a very faithful request. If she was still in the bed-and-breakfast business, could we reserve her home for Cornell's 2004 graduation weekend? It was a totally uncharacteristic move on my part. But the Holy Spirit said *write*, so I did.

When Sara called on Thursday, December 21, she apologized profusely for not responding sooner. She had misplaced my phone number. I was humbled by Sara's gracious invitation to extend her home to us when Lorraine graduated.

"If I'm still here, you're welcome to come," she said.

I told her about the diagnosis. *Did practice telling others really make it easier*, I wondered? Her words of compassion and understanding still ring in my ears. After I hung up, I received the timing of her phone call—exactly one week after hearing the original diagnosis from the gynecologist—as God's assurance I'd live to see Lorraine graduate. It was also the same day I met the stranger Helen after leaving the bakery. If God worked through people, and I knew He did, I hoped to be around for a whole lot more.

*Just keep walking by faith, Irene. I know where I am leading you.*

Since then, Sara had written a heartwarming note dated January 11: *I have been keeping you in my prayers since you told me. Why? Oh why is there so much cancer? I had hoped to offer you the bed and breakfast when you bring your daughter back to Ithaca for free . . . My prayers and thoughts are with you . . . Please stop by when you get to Ithaca,* the thoughtful message of this mother of eleven children concluded.

Common sense prevailed, however, and I stayed home this trip. With my energy level at rock bottom, an eight-hour round-trip car ride to Cornell and back would be foolhardy.

Lora called Saturday afternoon. She had cooked dinner for me. Lovingly prepared by the hands of a good friend, the last meal before surgery included her delicious stewed tomatoes and homemade macaroni and cheese. During dinner, Dana and I talked easily about "Aunt Lora's" kindness as we passed the sweet potatoes and baked chicken between us for second helpings.

"So are you okay with everything, Dana?" I asked, carefully leading into the meat of my query. "Dad will be at the hospital all day Tuesday, and I don't want you home by yourself. What do you think? Would you like to have someone here with you after school?

"I don't need anybody here. I can handle it, Mom. I'll be okay by myself," she replied tersely.

"Are you sure, honey? It will help to have somebody here to talk with," I answered patiently while silently I prayed. We discussed a very short list of names. Sadly, they all required an airplane ticket to arrive by Monday night.

"What about Lora? She understands," I suggested gingerly, chewing a mouthful of her tomatoes.

"No, that's okay, I'll be fine. Really."

What was a mother on the verge of surgery supposed to do?

Amos returned from Ithaca late in the evening with news of his meeting with Sara and a loaf of her fresh-baked zucchini bread.

The instructions for the required bowel prep required no solid foods for two full days before the operation and only clear liquids up to midnight of the day before, so I didn't get to taste any, but it sure smelled delicious. Amos also reported on Lorraine's arrival on her dorm floor.

"You should have heard them calling, 'Lorraine, Lorraine.' I know she felt good," Amos said with a smile. The warm welcome for his daughter obviously buoyed his spirits too.

By Sunday evening, I felt weary, weak from hunger and drained from emptying my intestines once more. With only one more full day at home before the hysterectomy, I began yet another countdown. Monday evening before the surgery evolved into a surreal, slow motion time. I finished packing my hospital bag and stayed clear of the kitchen. On a mission from God, steadfast Stephanie dropped by with a new bathrobe to wear in the hospital, a delicately scented candle, and a card from Miss Emily, a wise and young at heart eighty-year-old friend and counselor.

I relaxed in a soothing candlelit bath and deeply inhaled the delightful new fragrance. The aroma filled the bedroom and my psyche with sweetness like fresh-cut flowers. With the stereo softly playing in the background, I dimmed the lights, propped comfortably on several pillows, and opened Miss Emily's card.

### For the Night before Surgery

*O Lord, I know I had better do my praying now.*
*In the morning they will sedate me and tranquilize me*
*And anesthetize me and whisk me away in a fog.*
*I will see faces and hear voices*
*But they will blend and merge into a haze. So I pray.*
*I pray for the surgeon whose skill is so vital.*
*I pray for the nurses whose help is so important.*
*I pray for the anesthetist and all the support staff.*
*I know you work with and through them.*
*I pray for my loved ones who are anxious*
*And who feel so helpless waiting in that Family Lounge.*

*I pray for me.*
*I confess that I am anxious.*
*Surely it would be unnatural*
*Not to feel a knot of apprehension deep inside.*
*I want to be well and strong again.*
*I am not asking you to guarantee that, O Lord.*
*I know such things cannot be guaranteed*
*But I know you understand my wanting and you care.*

*So be with me even though I will be too far out of it to pray.*
*Be with those doctors and nurses*
*Even though they will be too busy to pray.*
*Now let me rest.*
*Somewhere one of the Psalmists said of you,*
*"He gives his loved ones sleep." Thank you, God, and I'll say*
*    "Goodnight" instead of Amen.*

The timely poem and thoughtful card touched my heart. Although it was late, I called Miss Em to say thanks. I also dialed Stephanie. I wanted nothing left undone. Although it was almost 10:30, Amos was still at work finishing a project since he planned to be at the hospital all day Tuesday. Resting comfortably, I had accomplished all that could be done. Now, I was ready for the next step, so I thought.

Dana knocked softly on the bedroom door. Without her usual bluster, she sat gingerly on the edge of the bed close to my extended legs. She looked dejected.

"How are you doing tonight, dolly?"

"I don't want you to have cancer, Mom."

I reached for her hand.

"Well, neither do I." We both laughed. We agreed so seldom.

"Seriously, Mom. I don't want you to have this surgery."

"Well, that makes two of us." And we both laughed again.

"Are you going to be all right, Dana? Would you like to have someone here with you tomorrow, after all?"

Sheepishly, she nodded in assent.

"No problem. Let's pray. I know God has someone in mind."

We held hands and bowed our heads. I always appreciate the privilege of hearing Dana's prayers. They are short and sweet and uncompromisingly to the point. When she finished, one name came to mind. Although it was nearly eleven o'clock, I reached for the phone, quickly dialed the familiar number, and explained this last-minute situation.

"No problem, Dana," I reported after the brief telephone conversation ended. "Lora will be here after school."

January 23 dawned clear and cold. The hospital admissions office expected me at 9:15 a.m. Since rush-hour traffic often backlogged early, we left a little before eight o'clock for the forty-minute drive into the city. In the Philadelphia region, hardly a day passes without news of another overturned, jack-knifed tractor-trailer truck creating havoc on the roadways. The last thing I needed was a traffic logjam. Nevertheless, at 8:50 not only were we at a standstill barely crawling through a sea of cars, we still had not crossed the Walt Whitman Bridge into the City of Brotherly Love.

I looked over at Amos. At the touch of a button, I reclined the seat and looked up through the sunroof at God's blue heaven. Hungry, weak, and growing agitated by the annoying traffic delay, I was certain this was not the mood I wanted to carry with me when I arrived at the hospital.

*Dear heavenly Father, you know all about this. You have this covered and completely under your control . . . just like all the rest of the stuff I've been dealing with. I've heard you, Lord. Having done all, stand. So it may look like I'm reclining in this car, but I'm standing, Lord. Standing on your promises to take care of me and get us safely to this hospital. Guide Amos, Lord. Get us there in peace, Lord. I know you can do it, so I'm saying thank you, Lord. In Jesus's name and on the authority of that name, I say Amen. Hallelujah!*

I opened my eyes just briefly enough to see Amos skillfully maneuver the car through traffic, taking indecent liberties to merge into the nearest lane to exit while still in New Jersey. The unfamiliar exit brought us to a quiet, tree-lined residential street. I had no idea where we were or how to get across the bridge. Thank God I wasn't driving. Fortunately, God endowed Amos with a sixth sense when it comes to finding his way out of unfamiliar territory. After a few minutes, he saw a sign for the bridge. Accelerating to reenter a road less traveled, we were soon on our way to Philadelphia.

"I'll have to remember that little detour," Amos remarked.

"Thank God," I responded.

We arrived at the busy hospital entrance around 9:39 by the Acura clock. The drive to the hospital normally required only forty minutes. Today, on a Tuesday morning, the same trip took nearly two hours to cover the distance. Go figure.

*Well now, Father. That wasn't normal. That was weird. I sure hope this trip wasn't a prelude to the remainder of this day.*

Then I remembered: I was talking to God using the wrong tone. *Forgive me, Lord. Yeah, I know. One moment at a time, Lord. One moment at a time. Stay on the moment-by-moment plan.*

After checking in at the hospital admissions office, an efficient woman directed us to the fourth-floor surgical-staging area. I waited only briefly before an attendant called me. She repeated my name, verifying the match on the hospital's identification wristband. She snapped the band securely around my wrist. Then she handed me a hospital gown and oversized green elastic footies.

"Are you nervous?" she asked.

"No," I replied, slowly drawing out the long vowel. "I'm praying."

Amos hugged me tightly before I climbed up on the gurney. A long, dimly lit corridor stretched endlessly ahead.

"I'm praying for you," he assured me as he quickly kissed dry lips.

The surgical nurse made me as comfortable as possible while I waited for the anesthesiologist. Another nurse thrust a clipboard at me with more authorization papers to sign. Then the surgeon appeared with some additional paperwork.

"The ones you signed before were misplaced or misfiled," she confessed.

"Does that mean I can still back out of this?" I asked jokingly as I signed the paperwork authorizing surgery once more.

The surgeon also discussed pain management. On our initial meeting back in December, I spoke openly about agonizing postoperative discomfort. Every surgery I've ever had left me writhing in excruciating pain. Whatever she could do to alleviate another painful aftermath got my unanimous vote. She highly recommended a self-administered system, the port for which would be inserted in my back at the outset of the surgical procedure. This would allow me to administer morphine at intervals I controlled, instead of the typical oral delivery of painkilling drugs every four to six hours.

Almost as an afterthought, the specialist mentioned the results of the MRI. "It's a good thing you had that done," she said. "The tumor is high in the cervix, the endocervix," she briefly explained.

The tumor's location was significant because the biopsy showed adenocarcinoma, that is, cancer cells from the uterus. This may have accounted for the initial confusion over the diagosis. HUP's philosophy was to remove the malignant growth surgically in the case of both cervical and uterine cancer.

A nurse who was part of my surgical team wheeled me into the surgical corridor. I could not enter the room immediately, however, because they weren't completely ready to begin. From my vantage point in the hallway, I saw one person scurrying busily, setting instruments on rolling tables, and another mopping the floor.

*Lord, I thank you for being here with me. Thank you for guiding the hands of all the people who will be working on me today. Thank you for those who are praying for me at this moment.*

It wasn't until the nurse rolled me into the sterile operating theater that the full impact of having reached the point of no return hit me squarely with its ultimate finality. They were removing my uterus today, and I was so glad: God gave me Lorraine and Dana. *I love those girls.* But I was also elated for another reason: while I liked being female, I sure wouldn't miss those messy, smelly monthly periods. No more accidentally stained clothing or soiled bed linens. I could forget about that aisle in the grocery store. I sat hunched over on the edge of the operating table. The surgical nurse swabbed my back and prepped me for the estimated three-hour radical hysterectomy: removal of the uterus and cervix, the fallopian tubes, ovaries, and some surrounding perimetrial tissues. As part of the surgical procedure, the surgeon would also dissect and remove some of the lymph nodes in my abdomen to check for the spread of disease. As the efficient team began their job, I not only thanked

God Almighty for making me a mother, but also for calling me His child, a cub of the Lion of Judah. Then, this daughter of the King of Glory started to hum: *In the shadow of his wings I will take refuge. In the shadow of His wings I will abide . . . until these trials, these present trials . . . until these calamities pass.* The last voice I heard came from one of the nurses who held my hand. "You won't be awake much longer."

⸺

When I awoke from the surgery, the first face I saw belonged to my surgeon. She stood to my right, and her blue eyes were smiling.

"You're doing fine," she said.

I could not speak. I turned my head slowly from side to side. Wide-eyed with wonder, I felt like I was seeing everything for the very first time. The clock on the wall to the left rendered the correct time, but was it morning or night? To the right, past the surgeon's head, the spacious recovery room contained several curtained areas where I supposed other patients lay. I noticed rows of supply cabinets. Two nurses, talking in hushed whispers, walked briskly past. I imagined myself as a newborn babe, and everything was new. I looked to the left, then to the surgeon on the right.

"I'm alive, Doc. Is everything all right?" Strangely, my own voice sounded unfamiliar.

"You came through fine. There were some complications, but we'll talk later," she said. "For now, just get some rest, then you'll be transferred up to your room," she ordered, gently patting my hand.

I closed and reopened my eyes. The surgeon had disappeared. Looking left again, then right, everything in the room had an amazingly sharp outline and clarity. Everything was new.

"I'm alive," I whispered.

*Thank you, Father. Thank you, Jesus. Thank you, Lord.*

Life in Christ is not the absence of trials and heartache or pain and suffering. It is knowing God and experiencing a profound gratitude for life itself. The Holy Spirit lives in me. God didn't have to wake me up after this surgery, but He did. Softly, I sang once more: *Jesus paid it all. All to Him I owe . . .*

# Chapter 7

## The Game Must Go On

☙ I press toward the mark for the prize of the high calling of God in Christ Jesus.

*Philippians 3:14*

Once vital signs stabilized, a friendly orderly wheeled me carefully into a waiting elevator for the short ride to the fourth floor of the hospital's Ravdin Wing. Rolled into Room 4024, I smiled. I wasn't so far gone not to notice the room's solitary bed. I experienced no physical pain whatsoever. Thank God for morphine.

*Oh, thank you, Lord Jesus. Heavenly Father, you know I appreciate this privacy. And I'm in no pain, Lord. No pain. Thank you, Lord.*

Transfer from the gurney to the bed raised the concept of "safe handling procedures" to a whole new level. After the nurse took the required care with the IV lines and the catheter tubing, I adjusted to the bed and new surroundings. The nurse poked and prodded, swiftly checking vital signs and the IV lines for the epidural to self-administer morphine. Proficient hands strapped hydraulic massagers on my legs. The incessant sound, motion, and pressure helped to visualize circulation to the lower extremities.

Once the nurse concluded her duties, she finally left me alone with a familiar old face.

"I love you," Amos said softly. He reached for my free hand and kissed my cheek.

"Ditto," I affirmed and squeezed his hand. "I love you too."

"Let's pray together," my weary husband suggested and bowed his head.

Amos sat in the straight-backed chair. He explained that complications required a urologist to assist in the operating room because scar tissue from prior abdominal surgeries obstructed the bowel and bladder. The extensive surgery had taken nearly eight hours, more than twice the estimated time.

"It was a good thing you had this surgery," he concluded.

I could only nod.

His good friend Bill kept him company in the surgical waiting room during the lengthy procedure.

"What a blessing. I didn't expect that," Amos said.

I could only nod. Then, I remembered.

"Dana? How's Dana. Did you call her and Lorraine?"

"I talked to Dana. She's fine. Lora came over. I'll call Lorraine when I get home."

I slowly nodded again and shifted to find a more comfortable position.

Dozing intermittently, I opened my eyes to see Amos sitting beside the bed.

"Are you watching me?" I asked. "You must be exhausted."

He could only nod.

"I'm going to stick around until the doctor shows up. Then I'll be headed back over the bridge."

The surgeon arrived with an entourage of four female residents. First, she introduced everyone, and then she examined the tender, swollen incision.

"Everything looks good," she assured me. Then she explained the reason for the surgery's complexity.

"You had a lot of scar tissue. There's a stent in your kidney, and we're going to leave the catheter in place once you're discharged," she said. The catheter eliminated the need to get in and out of bed to use the bathroom.

While I didn't understand everything she said, I still nodded. For the moment, moving my head like a bobbing-head doll worked for me.

"I'll see you tomorrow," she said with a gracious smile while patting my hand. "I want you to start walking tomorrow."

I nodded slowly and sighed.

*She wants me to walk, Lord. I barely have strength to nod, and she wants me to walk!*

Her suggestion unnerved me. *How can she even think I can walk down the hall when I can barely move in this bed,* I thought with some irritation.

After Amos left, I dozed in and out of consciousness. On a restricted diet of water and ice chips, I sipped and sucked, knowing this too shall pass. Day three without food was the least of my problems. Periodically tapping the button to release the morphine, I felt no pain, and I fully intended to keep it that way, praise God.

An orderly asked if I wanted to activate the overhead television set. I respectfully declined. I watch very little TV programming at home, so now was definitely not the time to start. Actually, even in a drug-induced state, I preferred the silence. Without the constant beckoning of the business telephone, I might actually get some modicum of rest in the postoperative phase. As the night wore on, I remained relatively pain free. The strange sensation of the reddish brown urine outflow caused some consternation, but I least I didn't have to get out of bed. At the moment, not walking anywhere worked just fine. Disturbing night sounds carried even behind the closed door. Muffled, anguished cries of women in pain down not-too-distant corridors were unmistakable throughout the night.

*Lord Jesus, help these women. Help them. Heaven help us all.*

In the early-morning hours before dawn, my thoughts turned to the freshman football player injured in a crippling tackle at a Penn State football game. The catastrophic collision in September 2000 left him paralyzed in a wheelchair. Told he would never walk again, this young man wasn't buying. Steadfast and immovable at his side, his father affirmed faith in God: his son would walk again. Before leaving for college, Adam Taliaferro lived within walking distance of my home. I've known his family casually since Adam and Lorraine attended first grade. The last time I saw Adam in person, his confident swagger across the shopping center parking lot had the distinctive mark of a determined young man with a bright future ahead.

"So are you all set for school? When do you leave?" I asked.

"In a couple of days," he answered with a broad smile. "Football practice starts early."

"God be with you and be careful," I replied.

*Watch over him, Lord. Keep him safe.*

Now, I remembered our last exchange and the prayer. While doctors insisted the odds were slim to none Adam would walk again, he took his first halting steps right before Christmas. So what was my problem?

The new nursing shift checked in around seven o'clock. The earlier reluctance to stand and place one foot in front of the other became a hope. Like the little engine that could, I entertained the thought that it *was* possible to walk today, after all. The surgeon strongly suggested it. Even if I only got as far as the door, I was willing to give it a try. Convinced that with God, all things are possible, I pushed the nurse's call button around ten o'clock that morning.

"I'd like to take a walk. My doctor said I should walk," I said when an aide poked her head inside the heavy wooden door.

"I'll have to get your nurse," she replied.

When the nurse on duty entered the room, she came directly to the bedside.

"So you're ready for a walk?"

"God willing, I'm going to try."

She immediately sprang into action, checking the IV lines and the catheter tubing. When she unplugged the pneumatic leg massagers and ripped the Velcro closures apart, my startle response ratcheted into high gear. My legs were hot and sweaty, but her next comment made me smile.

"Pretty toes," she said.

"Thanks," I replied, grateful for the decision to keep an appointment with Thom for a pedicure and manicure. Yes, I was going to get up, comb my hair, brush my teeth, go for a walk, and when I got back maybe make a few phone calls.

With all attachments secured, the able nurse adjusted the hospital bed and hoisted me up to a sitting position.

"Ooouch," I cried, painfully aware of the pressure on my tender, swollen belly.

The nurse helped me put the arm without the IV into the sleeve of the robe Stephanie gave me. I struggled from the edge of the bed and held the nurse's extended arm for support. Wincing, I stood hunched over and grabbed the IV pole. I certainly didn't want to fall.

*Help me, Jesus.*

"Steady now," the nurse cautioned. "Give yourself some morphine. That will help."

"This is tricky."

"You can do it."

With slow, baby steps, I dragged the rolling IV pole with my right hand and held the nurse's arm with my left. We made it through the wide doorway into the hallway. I was walking . . . praise the Lord Jesus!

As a volunteer chaplain, I had walked these same halls countless times visiting patients on the seventh floor of the Rhoads Wing. Knocking softly on the heavy wooden doors, I always entered a patient's room with the silent prayer,"Go ahead of me, Father," and He always did.

Now, I was the patient. The prayer and His answer were still the same.

"I'm okay," I told the nurse. "I can make it."

I inched to the nurses' station. One of the residents I'd met the night before recognized me as she rounded the corner.

"Is that you, Ms. Pace? I don't believe you're walking already. That's terrific," she said encouragingly.

"Praise the Lord," I responded with some measure of cheer.

This was just the boost I needed. At that very moment, I was contemplating turning back. After all, I didn't want to overdo it. Perfectly understandable, I rationalized. God had me walking. I wasn't going to put Him to the test by doing anything rash. Nonetheless, I turned the corner to the right. I was on a roll. Putting one foot in front of the other and pulling the pole took effort. Miraculously, I reached the end of the hallway.

I knew this rectangular layout like the back of my hand. As I slowly turned the corner, I clung to the IV pole like a spider on a wall. I was walking, but only barely. One step at a time, I praised my God for the strength to remain standing. I passed through the wide corridor at a snail's pace. Several open doors revealed patients who sat up in bed and others who looked unconscious. Determined to finish this marathon, I rounded the corner. As desolate as a stretch of barren desert, the wide corridor telescoped into view. This third leg of the journey seemed to extend for miles before the next turn leading back to my room. I stood stark still and gripped that pole so tight my knuckles turned white.

*Help me, Lord Jesus. Help me. Please don't let me fall down.*

I inched down the lengthening corridor. My life depended on dragging the pole. I walked by faith. My robe slipped from a slumping shoulder. *I must not fall.* If only I could get closer to the wall for added support. That's what I need . . . just a little more support. At just that moment, the orderly who brought my liquid breakfast tray emerged from a patient's room.

"Do you need some help?" she asked.

*Thank you, Jesus. Thank you. Thank you.*

"Oh yes, praise God. Walking is hard work," I responded gratefully.

She extended a strong arm, and I leaned hard, all the while expressing gratitude for God's perfect timing.

"I'll call your nurse when we get back," she said.

Safely back in the bed, nothing else mattered except getting some rest. No phone calls, no toothbrushing, no nothing. Exhausted, I pushed the button to release another dose of morphine. Amos brought me flowers that night, and I told him all about my eventful morning.

On the second afternoon, I awoke to the sound of a light tap on the door. A familiar face peered into the room. A trademark print wrap covering spiral twists adorned her head.

"Well, praise the Lord," I began. "Come on in here, girl," I beckoned this special visitor.

Ramona serves as volunteer coordinator of the hospital's pastoral care department. I first met her back in 1995 in one of the hospital's first-floor ladies rooms . . . a "divine appointment" if there ever was one. Orchestrated by God himself, just too many things had to line up in a very precise and specific sequence for our initial meeting to be just a chance encounter. During two years of volunteer work with cancer patients, I experienced many more divine appointments with Ramona. Each time we'd run into each other unexpectedly, we would invariably giggle like schoolgirls and hug like long-lost friends.

As a volunteer, I witnessed fear and terror in other's eyes at the mere mention of cancer. I saw grown men cry, and I cried with them. Between 1996 and 1998, I observed hundreds of cancer patients, principally those diagnosed with leukemia, lymphomas, and other blood-related cancers. Not everyone trusted Jesus Christ as Savior, and as the Lord who heals. Nonetheless, I came away with an unmistakable impression: those who cherished a time-tested relationship with the Lord Jesus seemed more resilient and hopeful because of their faith than those who lacked spiritual awareness and belief. They still had cancer, but it never diminished their hope. Believers in Christ Jesus consistently vocalized a steadfast faith in the Holy Spirit's power to heal and help them handle one of life's most difficult challenges. They seemed to cope better emotionally and psychologically than cancer patients without a spiritual anchor, and so did their families, I surmised. As a privileged insider to what cancer can and cannot do, I waved Ramona closer, warmly welcoming my former colleague in ministry.

As she approached the bed, a wonderful smile spread across her face. In the touch of her hand, I felt warmth and love emanating from the entire pastoral care team. This love, and the needs of countless patients, drew me to HUP week after week for two years straight. This love left little doubt HUP would be my first choice and only real option for cancer treatment. This love represented the best the Shepherd offers. Ramona's eyes reflected love's amazing power.

"I didn't want to wake you," she replied with a natural lilt in her soft voice.

"Are you kidding? I'm so glad to see you. Thank you for coming."

We laughed and reminisced. It was just like old times, and yet it was altogether new. Then, she prayed for me and hurried away to see other patients on the floor. Later that afternoon, an aide delivered a lovely, fresh-cut floral arrangement. The card was jointly signed "with love from Lisa, Denise, and Connie," Dana's art teacher and two of my neighbors. When Amos arrived with more flowers from Charlotte in Los Angeles, God's comfort enveloped me through the abundant blessing of friends who cared.

*Thank you, thank you, Father. All is well.*

By the third day, I sat in the reclining chair for over an hour, just staring out the window across a courtyard. Strength to walk around the floor's perimeter increased. I gained more momentum each day. With this moderate exercise and movement, a sponge bath with warm packaged cloths sufficed. But once the surgeon gave the okay on Day 4 to remove the IV lines tethered to my aching arm, more than anything I wanted to shower. The nurse brought towels and placed a white plastic chair outside the spacious stall in the adjoining bath.

"Just keep your back to the water flow," she cautioned.

Donning a shower cap and carefully adjusting the spray, I stepped inside and felt warm water pulsate against my skin. *Heaven must be like this*, I mused. Avoiding the incision while rinsing all the soap required far more energy than I imagined, however. By the time I stopped the water, stepped out, sat down, and partially dried myself, I was exhausted beyond belief. I looked at the bright red nurse's call button. I hesitated only momentarily, and then pulled the chord.

*I need help, Lord.*

During the next couple of days, I grew stronger, but bowel function had not returned. I needed to pass gas, but it just wasn't happening. Flatulence after abdominal surgery is normal. Expelling gassy accumulations in the intestinal tract indicates normal resumption of bowel function. By Saturday night, although I had not eaten any solid food in a week, I felt bloated and uncomfortable. In total desperation, I asked the aide who brought my liquid dinner for some prune juice. I took the drastic step of pouring about 1/4 teaspoon of the brown liquid into a four-ounce cup of apple juice. Prune juice always got me going. Clearly, something had to give.

I sipped less than half of the lukewarm mixture and alternated with clear water over the course of the evening. Later that night, I lived to regret it. The gas started around midnight. By midafternoon the next day, I experienced a full-blown case of the runs. When Amos and Dana arrived, I barely had energy to sit up. It was Super Bowl Sunday, and my two sports fans requested the television hookup.

"You don't want to miss the Super Bowl, Mom," Dana insisted.

"It will take your mind off how you're feeling," Amos chimed in as they unloaded a bag of snacks.

Amos took a seat in the oversized reclining chair near the window. Dana sat in the straight-back chair to the left of the bed. Sandwiched between the two—Amos flipping channels, and Dana munching from a supersized bag of chips—I faced the undeniable truth. I might have diarrhea, but the game must go on. By half time, I was weak and sore from repeated trips to the bathroom. At half time the Baltimore Ravens led the New York Giants, 3-0. My position: behind the eight ball!

During morning rounds, the surgeon raised my hopes by discussing discharge the next day, if normal bowel function returned. Well, once again, this wasn't what I called normal, but my bowels were working, no doubt about it. As the Super Bowl game progressed, I trekked to the bathroom repeatedly during the second quarter and long into the night. Weaker with every trip, I needed to drink something to avoid dehydration, but no sooner than I swallowed, the liquid flowed through me like a sieve.

The surgeon arrived with her entourage of eager residents early Monday morning around seven o'clock. I mentioned the persistent diarrhea. It didn't take a medical degree to see I wasn't at my level best, but she still gave me hope.

"Let's see how you do today since your stool is moving. It's okay to take some Imodium, and you can be on a regular diet now. If everything goes well after lunch, you can go home today," she said.

*Father, did you hear that? I can go home. Home. Oh, praise God! Home! Home to my own room. My own bed. Home! I'm going home today.*

"Praise the Lord, Doc," I affirmed with pure joy.

After she and the other residents left, I reached for the phone and called Amos. I hoped to share this welcome news before he left for work.

"Thank God. That's wonderful. What time should I come for you?" he asked.

"Doc said after lunch," I replied quickly, mentally calculating the departure time. "I'm coming home."

The breakfast tray with its dome-covered plate looked unappetizing. I wasn't as hungry as I thought, even after more than a week without solid food. I ate the banana and the muffin, but the bland bowl of oatmeal just didn't get any votes. As the morning progressed, I freshened up and combed my hair. I was going home. Amos arrived shortly after lunch and ate the chicken, broccoli, and mashed potatoes, which I barely touched. I wasn't hungry. I was going home. Even with the Imodium, the diarrhea persisted into the early afternoon, but it didn't matter. Nothing mattered. I was going home.

Dressed and ready for discharge, I dozed into the late afternoon, and so did Amos. The doctor was later than I thought she would be. Didn't she say "after lunch"?

Shortly before five o'clock, the doctor's gentle knock and entrance signaled the beginning of the end of my seven-day hospital stay.

"How are you feeling?" she asked. Poised to listen attentively, her residents leaned forward.

"I'm ready to go, Doc. I'll be fine."

"Then we'll get the discharge papers ready and get you some instructions for the catheter bag and how to change it," she replied. "I'll want to see you in about a week." I could expect a call from her office to schedule a follow-up appointment to check the incision.

*It is finished, Father. I'm going home.*

The surgeon moved closer.

"You've done well," she said.

Eyeball to eyeball, I nodded and smiled. From my beside perch with my legs dangling to the floor, I saw a *woman* doctor. My surgeon sidestepped the catheter bag and hugged me. Her unexpected gesture warmed my heart. The touch of her arm around my shoulders felt awkward and unmistakably tender at the same time. *This consummate professional and skilled surgeon cared.*

"Thank you, Doc," I said. "Learn as much as you can, so you can help somebody," I advised the four female residents.

Packed and ready, I could finally leave the hospital. The nurse returned with discharge instructions, along with a new catheter bag and plastic tubing.

"Do you have a Depend? Just in case," I implored with a whisper.

She returned with the largest adult diaper I have ever seen. Having lost over ten pounds in seven days, I needed a smaller size, but this was not the time or place to be choosy. I was going home. An orderly wheeled the required wheelchair to the bedside.

Bundled in an oversized down stadium jacket, I gingerly maneuvered for maximum comfort.

"Watch the bag," I urged, hoping to avoid accidentally bumping the catheter bag or tubing.

Back in the spacious hospital lobby, Amos fished for his parking stub and waited for the valet to return his car.

"You're going home," Amos's words sounded as smooth as silk. I tightly squeezed his hand. "Praise God, honey. Praise the Lord."

Traffic flowed smoothly during the post-rush-hour drive back home to New Jersey. Amos's Acura seemed to glide across the blacktop with only an occasional and very disconcerting bump.

"Easy now," I pleaded, supporting my abdomen under the bulky green coat.

I watched the garage door's slow ascent as Amos pulled into the driveway.

"I'm home, Amos. I'm back home."

I felt slight pain while sitting, but now it was time to stand.

Amos carefully eased me from the car. Slow and steady, we walked arm in arm through the garage toward the kitchen door.

Struggling inside, I saw Dana standing next to the kitchen table. She appeared puzzled, but to tell the truth, I was in no shape to discern the look on her face. Tears clouded my vision.

"Happy birthday, Dana," I said.

I *so* wanted to sound cheery. An eternal optimist, I needed to inject an uplifting note into this homecoming. The discomfort in my belly and the oncoming rush of overflowing tears belied the vocal veneer, however. Besides, Dana's keen insight was legendary. She was sure to penetrate my flimsy ruse. I reached for my dear daughter and held her tight.

"I'm home, Dana. I'm back home."

# Chapter 8

## The Catheter

**⛌ I love the Lord, because he hath heard my voice . . . therefore I will call upon him as long as I live.**

*Psalm 116:1-2*

The first Thursday in February marked my first excursion to the downstairs level of my home in eleven days. The return to the kitchen matched the same number of days the Israelites needed to reach the Promised Land, *if* they had taken the direct route instead of the forty-year journey. The night the surgeon discharged me from the hospital, I struggled to climb the six stairs leading to the upstairs hallway. I shuffled into the bedroom, all the while leaning heavily on Amos's strong arm. With two feet on each step, the laborious ascent only strengthened my resolve: once upstairs, I would not venture back down before the next scheduled visit to the hospital unless the house was on fire.

*I know you're with me every step of the way, Lord.*

To conserve precious strength and allow total freedom from any concern about household chores, I promised myself this eleven-day upstairs sabbatical. Healing takes time, and I had time to spare. No energy, but plenty of time.

*Holy Spirit, I know you have power to keep your word. Please help Dana to adjust.*

While Amos went to the grocery store pharmacy to fill prescriptions, Dana appeared clearly uncomfortable in the nurse's aid role. I couldn't use my own bathroom because the pungent smell of bleach permeated the small enclosed area.

"Dad's been cleaning up, Mom," Dana explained curtly.

With the catheter bag in tow, Dana help me to shuffle back into the hallway to use her bathroom. I was so weak I could barely sit down on the toilet without reaching back for the seat cover with one hand and holding Dana's arm with the other. She helped me the best she knew how. I sat doubled over on the stool when suddenly an explosive heave erupted from the depths of my belly. There was no time or energy to stand. Waves of slimy green puke splashed into the adjacent bathtub while the putrid odor filled our nostrils. Today, January 29, marked Dana's milestone birthday, not exactly the "sweet sixteen" she envisioned.

"Mom! Are you all right? Where's Dad? Are you all right?" Dana asked, her frenzied, wild eyes staring.

I looked hopelessly into her frantic eyes. For the past eight days, my dry, cracked lips had not touched even a scrap of solid food until this morning. Bouts of diarrhea for the past forty-eight hours had surely drained me dry. What more could possibly be left behind?

"At least I didn't vomit on the floor," I said wanly, an effort to console us both.

Now, almost two weeks later, I recalled events etched indelibly in my mind while preparing to leave for the first follow-up visit to the hospital. Dana's sixteenth birthday was *some* party; but now it was time for a maiden voyage downstairs and some real celebrating. First, the urologist would remove the catheter from my bladder. Next, the surgeon planned to remove the staples securing the incision. I had a big day ahead and a big God to help me through it.

Amos opted to work early that morning and planned to return around 11:30. Before he left, my neighbor Linda arrived to keep me company.

"Hi there," she called, entering the bedroom with a wave and a smile. "Nice furniture," this interior designer observed.

I embraced my friend with a grateful hug. Even though it had been fifteen days since the operation, I still appreciated the "room service" and thoroughly enjoyed whatever company happened by for an "upstairs" visit.

"I'm so glad you could come, Linda," I said.

She dismissed my gratitude with a wave and a shrug. "No problem," she insisted. "You've lost weight," she observed.

Even a casual observer could detect these navy nylon pants looked baggy at the hipline, but I didn't care. I was alive and able to braid my hair in two cornrows and apply cocoa foundation and plum lipstick. I laughed with Linda about the days and nights spent upstairs. We compared notes on the lives of our daughters, both aged sixteen. All was well. In about sixty minutes or so, I would be relieved of this catheter tube between my legs. When I first came home, a sickly, blood-clotted burgundy-colored urine filled the bag. With time, the color of the continual flow gradually changed to reddish yellow.

*I will never take the ability to urinate for granted again, Father God. Thank you for the pale golden hue, Lord Jesus.*

Emptying the bag's contents into the commode took some practice, but after today, the doctor would pull the plug on this chapter.

*Glory hallelujah! Praise your holy name, Lord.*

When we arrived at the hospital entrance, Amos waited impatiently for one of the blue-jacketed parking attendants. Several empty wheelchairs sat in disorganized array in the busy curbside area adjacent to the huge revolving door.

"Need a ride, Miss Daisy," he joked easily, opening the door to help me from the car.

The incision was still tender, and the weight of the catheter bag strapped to my calf under my pants made me skittish. I struggled from the low car seat as carefully as possible and eased into the rolling chair. *Today the urologist would remove this thing.* The mere thought evoked visions of cartwheels. Waiting over two hours for the procedure to begin significantly cooled my heels, however. Amos intermittently watched television, dozed, or flipped disinterestedly through a stack of outdated magazines. I was simply hungry and exhausted from futile attempts to find some small comfort on the hard waiting room chair. Half naked in a wrinkled hospital gown, I used my heavy wool coat like a blanket. With the catheter bag strapped to my leg, I felt tethered like a dog on a leash. Two patients ahead of me sought the same release. While I didn't know what to expect, it would not be long now.

At long last someone called me for the 12:30 appointment with destiny. Escorting me into the examination room, the weary-eyed nursing assistant apologized for the delay. A six-year-old child needed extensive emergency treatment, she explained. I glanced at the large round clock on the wall. It was 2:40.

Once inside, the attending nurse invited me to sit on the edge of a long horizontal table which practically spanned the entire length of the room. Only a thin white sheet separated my bare derrière from the table's cold, hard surface. She flipped expertly through my bulging medical charts. Then the young woman rolled a cart full of medical apparatus in front of the table to take vital signs. My thin legs dangled casually. After seven days in the hospital following surgery, I was accustomed to the routine procedures. Pulse . . . I stuck the index finger in the electronic gizmo. Temperature . . . she poked the electronic gadget in the right ear. Blood pressure . . . the black nylon cuff tightened around a flabby upper arm. I remained completely unfazed until she left the room and returned quickly with a barium milkshake.

"Drink this," she directed, handing me a white Styrofoam cup. "This will help show us your internal organs," she added.

*Not again, Lord. I hate this stuff.*

I obediently downed the cool, thick milky white liquid. It tasted like watery vanilla yogurt. With each swallow, I rolled my eyes heavenward, then I returned the empty cup with wide-eyed curiosity. This was the first time I had worn a catheter, and quite frankly, I had some honest questions about its removal.

"You can lie back down now," she said.

"Just what *exactly* is going to happen?" I asked with polite nonchalance, resting uneasily on the cold, hard surface. The youthful attendant dutifully supported my knees to ease any back strain. I looked at her face expectantly.

With an animation that surprised me, she explained in vivid detail how I was about to take a little ride. This was no ordinary table: it rotated from the horizontal to the vertical axis at the touch of a button. The control panel remained safely out of my reach behind a smoked glass window in an adjacent room. The barium liquid would highlight a red contrast dye the doctor would inject into blue-green veins. Reaching up, the nurse touched a two-by-three-foot screen positioned about four feet above my head.

"The projection screen shows your organs at work," she said. "You'll be able to see the catheter, your bladder, even the stent in your kidney once the dye gets in your bloodstream," she added.

"I didn't notice that before," I said, looking dubiously at the smooth white surface and shifting uncomfortably.

"It moves too," the nurse said with a smile.

I looked above once more.

After the table rotated to a standing position, the doctor would remove the tubing and then I would urinate, she concluded. I strained to get the exact mental picture in sharp focus.

"How long have you had the catheter?" she asked.

"I had surgery January 23. It's been almost two weeks now," I replied.

"Then you shouldn't have any problem at all," she assured, patting my arm. Because doctors inserted the catheter over a week ago, I should urinate quite easily if the bladder had healed, she continued. Two weeks is generally sufficient time for healing. If not, reinsertion was the only option. While the stainless steel stent in the kidney would remain in place for another six weeks, there was really no need to worry about a thing.

It sounded simple enough, but like many things medical, what happens in actual practice often differs radically from the textbook explanation. Sometimes, being naturally curious has its drawbacks. For now, at least, I knew *something*. After starting an IV in my right arm, the attendant placed lightweight black nylon straps across my chest and torso, securing my upper body firmly to the table. Next, I heard the smooth sound of a quiet motor as the nurse lowered the movable screen to within a foot of my chest and pelvis. At the touch of a button, she raised the screen to the original position.

"All set now," she said cheerfully. "The doctor will be ready in just a few minutes. Any more questions?"

I shook my head slowly from side to side. She left me alone to ponder the inevitable.

*I'm sure glad you're with me. Thank you, Lord, for getting me through this. Please let me pee when this is over. Lord, I know you're here.*

Now that I was completely prepped, the doctor made her entrance. Of medium height and build, her Indian accent had a soothing lilt. Straight dark hair framed the gentle face of a woman in her mid-forties. Her eyes and friendly smile exuded kindness.

"So how are you doing?" she asked, touching my arm to examine the IV.

"I'll be better when I get this out," I responded in reference to both the IV and the catheter.

"It won't be long now," the doctor assured, continuing the flow of small talk.

She checked the position of the overhead screen and started the injection process. The red dye moved quickly through my veins because in seconds I experienced a warm sensation in my bladder. With the light dimmed, I could see the outline of internal organs on the illuminated screen above me. Safe and secure behind the glass window, the assistant activated dials to start the vertical rotation of the nine-foot table and lower the attached screen. Slowly I felt myself lifting from a prone to a standing position like a lifeless marionette come to life.

*Help me now, Lord. Help me!*

Once on the vertical axis, I hoped and prayed the sheer force of gravity would not overtake me. Wide-eyed and unsteady, I felt like a cartoon character on the verge of falling facedown. Only these flimsy black straps restrained me from lunging forward headlong. Before I could think about my next move, the doctor returned with a crazy suggestion and a bizarre move of her own.

"Spread your legs," she commanded. "That will steady you."

"Huh?" I murmured in utter disbelief. As soon as I obeyed one order, she barked out another.

*My Jesus!*

"Hold this," she spoke firmly, thrusting a long plastic container between my legs. It looked like a quart-sized milk carton without the top. "Squeeze your legs. That will hold it."

*Lord Jesus!*

"Now when I pull this out, you'll be able to pee in the cup. Just relax now," she intoned in the ultimate oxymoron. In her same soothing voice, she instructed her assistant to turn on the water in a nearby sink.

*What's happening, Lord?*

Then, she yanked that catheter from my insides with the studied and practiced force of a bullfighter cracking a whip. It was over and out in the blink of an eye.

I was stunned! My mind heard the echoes of the old *Rawhide* series theme song. I wasn't hurting. In fact, I didn't feel a thing . . . it all happened so fast. Now I was supposed to urinate while standing strapped to the table with a milk carton between my legs.

*Were they kidding or crazy*, I wondered.

*Lord Jesus, you know I can't do this.*

The last time I tried to urinate while standing I was about six years old near some bushes across the street from Chicago's Buckingham Fountain in Grant Park. When I ended up with wet shoes and socks, I quickly surmised vertical urination was definitely for boys. Sandwiched between the moving table and the projection screen, I was trapped in a time warp somewhere in 1957. It was a defining moment. I might not have a uterus, but that didn't mean I could pee like a man.

I stood strapped in the vertical position for what seemed like an eternity (hospital time is quite different from *regular* time). I wanted desperately to relax and let it flow, but nothing came out. Not one golden yellow drop. I could see the outline of a bloated bladder on the illuminated white screen.

"You can do it," the soothing voice intoned.

*Lord, help me. This is crazy. Lord, have mercy on me!*

The doctor's repeated enticements to urge and coax bladder release continued incessantly, without success. After five *hospital* minutes, she mercifully relented.

"Turn the water off," she instructed her trusty assistant.

"As soon as you urinate, I'll be back to check on you," the doctor's pleasant voice assured me. Then, she gathered some papers and left the room.

"Relax," her accomplice suggested with a shrug as she removed the milk carton.

"What just happened? What was the water for?" I asked, a weak attempt to divert attention from my embarrassment and humiliation.

"Sometimes the sound of water helps you to go," she explained vaguely. "Maybe you would do better on the toilet," she suggested.

*The toilet? Lord, have mercy. Did she say there's a toilet?*

"The toilet!" I asked incredulously. I was completely dumbfounded.

She disappeared again briefly to push controls that slowly returned me to the horizontal plane. After unbuckling the restraining straps, the young assistant held a shallow oblong container in her hand. I struggled to sit upright.

"Why don't you try in the bathroom right here . . . just pee in this," she said, handing me a pink receptacle. "I have to check your urine output," she said dryly.

As soon as I stood up, the irrepressible urge took center stage and total control. Modestly covering exposed buttocks with the flimsy cotton gown, I hobbled dejectedly toward the bathroom. I sat down and immediately released the unstoppable flood. Warm urine splashed all over my hand. I was mortified.

*If I had another option, Lord, why didn't they tell me sooner?*

Stacks of paper towels and boxes of gauze bandages completely filled the bathroom sink. What a time to add insult to injury. I couldn't even wash my hands. I balled up the flimsy hospital gown and dumped it into the soiled linen hamper before leaving the dressing area. Amos waited patiently with the wheelchair for the next ride to yet another exam room. The cheerful receptionist greeted us warmly. This time, the familiar and compassionate surgeon removed the staples from the incision without any delay.

"You need to start walking," my surgeon gently admonished as Amos helped me settle into the wheelchair.

"I will," I nodded wearily. "Just not today."

Amos rolled me expertly through the hospital's winding corridors. I'd had a very long day, I realized with resignation, and it wasn't over yet as I braced for the forty-minute ride back home.

Memories of the day's events filled my mind. It was the first time I had ventured downstairs and out of the house in nearly two weeks. I was exhausted. Now, as I leaned against the kitchen door preparing mentally to maneuver the stairs, Dana bounded down.

"Hi, Mom," she said exuberantly. "I see you got rid of your latest fashion accessory," she quipped, her flippant reference to the catheter bag.

I smiled, sighed deeply, and moved toward the banister to steady myself before ascending the stairs.

*Lord, please help all teenagers . . . everywhere.*

Though tired, I showered sumptuously, lathering, splashing, and soaping again. Hot tears flowed freely in the warm, cascading spray. My chest heaved as the overhead downpour drenched my back. The catheter episode was over . . . finished.

*Hallelujah! Thank you, Jesus!*

Showering for the first time without the catheter felt like a caged bird suddenly freed. I will never again take the ability to urinate for granted. I resisted the temptation to turn around. Instead, I stood with my back to the water, careful to avoid accidentally touching the abdominal wound.

*Thank you, Jesus. Thank you, Jesus. Thank you, Jesus. We made it, Lord! Thanks for being with me just like you said you would.*

I lavishly massaged lotion all over my body, taking special care to avoid my swollen abdomen. Wounded in more ways than one, I embraced the precious freedom of my catheter-free status and the healing power of the fleeting moment. Because none of my underwear fit, I slipped into a pair of Amos's wrinkled cotton boxer shorts and pulled a white cotton tee shirt over my head. The worn sheets felt familiar, comfortable. I was back home again in my very own bed.

"Ready to eat something?" Amos called from the kitchen. "I'm coming up."

*I praise you, Lord, for that wonderful man.*

I eyed the tray with gratitude. I needed to regain fifteen pounds, much-needed weight lost since the surgery. While I ate, Amos joked that my normally healthy appetite was returning with a true passion.

"Do you want any dessert?" he asked.

All I wanted now was sweet dreams. After brushing my teeth, I hunkered down for some long-awaited rest. I dozed in and out of consciousness.

I got up to use the bathroom, and then I slipped back into bed wearing nothing but my birthday suit and diamond ring. I turned over in bed, but Amos wasn't there. *Was I dreaming?* Naked, I shopped in a crowded mall until I found Victoria's Secret and started browsing the lingerie tables. I couldn't find what I wanted.

*This is surreal. Who took my robe and slippers?*

"Can I help you?" asked a sales clerk dressed in a stylish black *pants suit. A long yellow crime scene tape circled her waist like a belt. She seemed nonplused to observe me naked as a jaybird.*

"I'm just looking," *I replied nonchalantly.*

*I approached another table piled high with satin panties. I still couldn't find the right pair.*

*"Look . . . there," I directed, pointing to some lacy black fabric sitting on the counter behind the cash register. "Yes, that's just what I was looking for."*

Amos appeared out of nowhere. "Just checking on you," he said, peering down on me. Then he disappeared. Was I dreaming?

*The woman in the black suit handed me the silkiest, sexiest, laciest, most expensive black panties in the store . . . size small.*

Nothing is too hard for God.

*"They're called tangas," she explained.*

*To my utter amazement, I realized I'd forgotten my handbag . . . no money, no checkbook, no credit card.*

With God, all things are possible.

*I could not afford the lacy lingerie. But I certainly couldn't afford to leave the store without them.*

# Chapter 9

## Is There a Nurse in the House?

🔑 **The Lord is my shepherd; I shall not want.**

*Psalm 23:1*

One week after the doctor yanked the catheter from my bladder, I received a special delivery package shortly after 10:30 that Thursday morning. Seated at the dining room table, I chatted easily with my good friend Michele who had dropped by to see if I needed anything.

"You look good," she said, raising her teacup.

"Praise the Lord," I replied, smiling broadly. "It's the Lord's doing. Plus, you know I'm just taking one day at a time."

"Have you already eaten breakfast?" she asked.

"I'm almost ready for my second breakfast," I joked.

In fact, once my appetite returned full force, I ate smaller, high-protein meals and snacked on fruits, vegetables, and nuts about five or six times each day. Generous neighbors and home-cooking friends did their part and more to ensure my family and I ate regular, nutritious dinners.

"You should look in the refrigerator. We're eating better than when I was shopping and cooking," I quipped.

With frequent visits from friends and plenty of food and rest, each day I grew stronger in preparation for chemotherapy, the next phase of cancer treatment.

As Michele and I talked, I heard Amos upstairs getting dressed for work. When the doorbell rang, he was just on his way downstairs. It was Gina, our neighborhood FedEx woman, with a special delivery package just for me. A big red sticker affixed to the medium-sized brown corrugated box got my attention: Keep refrigerated. DO NOT FREEZE.

I directed Michele to find a small utility knife in the kitchen, and together we opened the package. Inside, a white Styrofoam cooler rested on green foam peanuts.

"What's this?" I wondered aloud. "Oh, I know. They told me this would be coming," I recalled.

When the surgeon checked the incision the week before, she mentioned the need to build red blood cells in preparation for chemotherapy treatments. She prescribed weekly injections of Procrit, the same drug administered back in December at the first oncologist's office. I'd seen television commercials for Procrit many times. One advertisement portrayed an elderly man who needed energy to shop for his grandson's "big boy" bed. While the commercial's voice-over enumerates the drug's mild side effects, the happy grandfather omits a very important detail that surfaced in a telephone conversation with one of the nurses from my surgeon's office a few days before the FedEx package arrived.

"The medication will be shipped directly to your house," the nurse said. "Do you know a nurse who can help you?" she asked.

Actually, I knew several nurses personally. "Why do you ask?"

"You'll need someone to show you how to inject yourself," she answered.

*What! Lord, that guy on TV never said anything about that!*

"I'm supposed to inject myself?" I responded weakly, my voice barely audible.

When our conversation ended, I clicked the cordless phone, confident I would cross that bridge only when I came to it . . . no sooner.

*Jesus, will you please direct me to the nurse you have in mind? I didn't know I had to inject myself. I had no idea I needed a nurse, Lord.*

What I didn't know could fill volumes, it appeared. Today's entry would be one for the books!

Michele struggled valiantly to remove the cooler from the outer box. Inside, a small plastic zip-lock bag contained several pale yellow disposable gloves, four packets of alcohol swipes, and four syringes. I opened a small white box and found four glass vials, about an inch high. A small bright red plastic container prominently featured the ominous poison symbol. The word "contaminated" stood out in bold black letters.

"Hmmmm," Michele mused, releasing her breath.

I asked her to put the box with the vials in the refrigerator while I reached for a large envelope resting inside the empty box. I gingerly opened it. Unblinking eyes riveted from the cost of the medication to a shocking illustration for its use. The four-week supply of Procrit cost $3,200 . . . $800 a pop! One look at the crude drawing, and I knew I was in *big trouble*. Stark black outlines—the front and back contours of a woman's body—diminished all other print. Randomly scattered dots along the arms, thighs, abdomen, and buttocks represented unmistakable potential injection sites. The pocked body image looked like a target practice sheet. Unfortunately, the gun must have been loaded with buckshot.

CHANGE INJECTION SITE EVERYTIME YOU
INJECT. REFER TO DIAGRAM BELOW. AREAS
COLORED IN GRAY ARE ACCEPTABLE
INJECTION SITES.

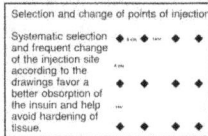

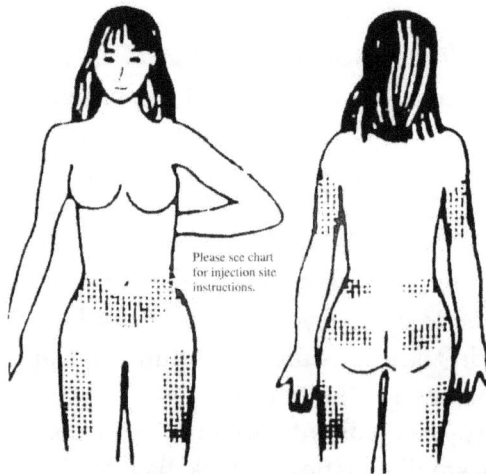

Selection and change of points of injection

Systematic selection and frequent change of the injection site according to the drawings favor a better obsorption of the insuin and help avoid hardening of tissue.

Please see chart for injection site instructions.

Michele returned from the kitchen and scrutinized my face intently. "Are you okay?" she asked.

"Yeah," I responded blankly as I quickly folded the papers and stuffed them back into the envelope. Now I needed time to recover from this special delivery. Placed between our teacups, the white envelope represented an unwelcome guest at the dining table.

*You have to take care of this, Lord. I cannot do it. I cast the care on you. I just can't think about this right now. You've got this. I know you've got this! Thank you, Father. Thank you for being with me, just like you said.*

I sipped tepid tea. The rolling floodwaters sounded closer than I was ready or willing to think about at this moment. I needed protection from the ravages of chemotherapy. But who could help me? The names of several nurses I knew came to mind.

*Lord God, please direct me to the right one. Self-injection? Lord, have mercy!*

After Michele left, I headed upstairs to rest. As I lay in bed, I thought about one of the standard queries on any medical history questionnaire, namely, "How many surgeries?" The vertical ten-inch wound, still tender and swollen, traversed the length of my abdomen from the navel to about three inches into the pubic area. I wouldn't be doing any sit-ups for a while. I was long past the notion of ever wearing a bikini.

Now that I could freely venture downstairs, I planned my trips carefully. Peering in the refrigerator, I could choose milk or juice, but I didn't have the physical strength to lift the gallon jugs. I admired the beautiful potted plants and exquisite floral designs friends had sent to cheer me, but I just couldn't lift them or carry the watering can to perk them up.

Rather than focus on my limitations, I made a conscious commitment to accentuate the positive. Walking downstairs, out the front door and taking baby steps, I slowly made it from the door to the end of the gravel driveway—about thirty-five feet. By the end of the week, I gained the strength to walk from the front door to the *nearest* corner. In earlier days, I thought nothing of the ten-to twenty-second walk to the corner. These days, up and back required all of ten minutes. The first time I ventured to the farthest corner from my house, I reached the milestone destination and clung to the light pole like white on rice. *Déjà vu.* Turning, I watched the familiar street stretch and lengthen with the same telescopic lens effect I experienced in the hospital corridor the day after surgery. It was only by the grace of God I returned home without collapsing in the middle of the street.

That night I called two nurses who share the same first name. Both attended Asbury United Methodist Church. Neither one was home, but in the calmest voice I could manage, I left the same urgent message on their respective answering machines: call me as soon as you get a chance.

*Whoever calls me back first, Lord. That's the one.*

Late the next evening, Rosolyn returned my call. We exchanged pleasantries, and thanks to what I learned from Dana, I quickly got to the point.

"I need your help, Ros. I need a nurse to show me how to inject this Procrit," I explained.

"No problem. You know I'm happy to do it," she responded. "When should I come?"

The drug required weekly injections. Ros, a full-time nurse coordinator in a local public school system, asked if Sunday after worship service would work for me.

"That would be great," I replied gratefully.

True to her word, Ros rang the doorbell on Sunday, February 18. The vaulted ceiling in the foyer was much too low for the high praise we gave our heavenly Father.

"You look wonderful," she affirmed.

"It's the Lord's doing," I replied.

I ushered her upstairs to the master bedroom where I had laid out the paraphernalia: a pair of disposable gloves, a packet of alcohol swabs, the syringe, and a forty-thousand-unit vial of Procrit.

"You're all set," she said.

*Not exactly*, I thought to myself, remembering the terrible sting of the first injection in December.

"So how do you do this, Ros?" I ventured, unfolding the illustration with the projected injection sites for the first time since that fateful day Michele and I opened the box. "What do I do?"

"What do you mean?" Ros asked with a puzzled look on her face. "I'm going to inject you. I'm your nurse. You don't have to worry about injecting yourself. I'll be your private duty nurse. I'll be here every week."

*Oh, dear Lord! Thank you, Lord. I knew I could trust you to take care of this.*

"Oh, Ros. Are you serious? That would be wonderful. I asked God to help me with this. I knew I couldn't do it," I gushed.

"No problem."

She opened her black bag and pulled out a stethoscope, blood pressure cuff, and a small reference book on prescription drugs. Ros wrote my name, address, and phone number on a blue index card, and then noted the date, the blood pressure reading, and the arm she would inject first.

"We'll alternate arms, first left, then right, so you won't get sore."

*A private duty nurse, Lord. You are awesome!*

Ros swabbed my arm, filled the syringe, and lightly tapped the needle to release any air bubbles.

"Don't want that," she advised. Sensing the tension, she simply said, "Relax."

"It hurt so bad before. I just stung like fire," I said.

"This won't hurt a bit," she assured me.

Lo and behold, it didn't. Afterward, I suggested a brief walk to the nearest corner. I glanced wistfully past the corner, and Ros encouraged me to give it a try.

"You can make it, Irene."

Arm in arm, we rounded the curve. Step by precious step, we walked to the first mailbox on the next block, turned around, and walked back home. Her encouraging visit marked the first time in nearly six weeks that, on foot at least, I'd ventured further than one hundred feet from the front door without the fear of falling down.

For the next eight weeks, nurse Ros kept her word. Only twice did she call a substitute. The other nurse named Roslyn filled in one week and brought her mother Jackie. The three of us shared our hope in Christ during a joyful visit in my bedroom. Another week, I carried all the paraphernalia to Sunday worship service. This time God placed nurse Gina on duty. This angel of mercy prepped me for the injection in a private room after service ended. I received seamless private duty nursing care. God's hand never left the helm.

*The Lord is my Shepherd. I shall not want.*

At no time did *any* need go unmet.

Not any of Dana's needs: On the night of the sophomore cotillion, the Divine Order Ministry team—three close friends I'd known for several years—transformed themselves into Christian Merry Maids.

"We're servants. That's all," Betty quipped as she cleaned the kitchen. Upstairs, Marty ironed a tablecloth, while Wanda ran the vacuum.

Michele stopped by the local florist, where some of my neighbors worked as floral designers. She delivered a dazzling floral arrangement for the dining room table and placed the boutonnière for Dana's boyfriend in the refrigerator. She even transported Dana to and from the hair salon and paid for her manicure. God also sent willing chauffeurs: Mamie drove Dana to weekly voice lessons; Donna transported her to art lessons; and Carolyn, bless her heart, volunteered to awaken at the crack of dawn to periodically drive Dana to school for her 6:50 chemistry class.

Not any of Lorraine's needs: Sight unseen, Lockheed Martin offered her a summer internship after receiving her resume via email before she returned to Cornell in January. And in February, Amos and I fell to our knees and praised God for seeing us through the first year of college tuition payments, paid in full! Lorraine came home for spring break in March. I barely blinked and she was gone.

Not any of Amos's needs: He had a job fifteen minutes away from home. The higher-ups at this job showed compassion for his time away from work to accompany me on numerous doctor visits and at treatment sessions. He sometimes worked until two or three in the morning to complete his work assignments, but God brought him through too. He owned a business where faithful clients waited patiently for merchandise deliveries. And God surrounded him with supportive colleagues at work and compassionate caregivers at home.

And certainly not any of my needs: God sent generous friends with delicious, home-cooked meals and delectable desserts with regularity. Missionary Marcy, a poet and friend from Asbury United Methodist Church, unloaded bags of groceries, toiletries, and laundry detergent one Saturday, and then cleaned the house as if it were her own. My neighbor Denise insisted I forget about the laundry and walked to the corner with me one sunny afternoon. Even at my snail's pace, it was much more fun to walk arm-in-arm with a friend than worry about falling in the street alone.

Asbury's Children's Church leaders Joann and Greg organized a get-well card project for children age three to twelve. In early February, and again in mid-March, the mailman delivered a large envelope brimming with handmade cards and handwritten notes. Each message conveyed love and encouragement. Although I received over two hundred cards and letters from well-wishing friends and concerned relatives around the country, the children's love notes left the most profound impression of the Shepherd's great tenderness. The message from ten-year-old Thea touched my heart.

She wrote: *"I hope that this letter is making you fill up with joy, and that the joy is heeling you alot . . . please don't be sick forever. If it is a little flew thing don't worry about it becuase it will probly go away soon . . . So keep on prayin and you won't fel a sick thing or organ in your body [sic]."*

Tommy wrote "WE MISS YOU" in big red letters. The message inside his card struck a sweet-sounding chord.

WE MISS
YOU

Asbury wants
you to know that
we miss you. Church
is borring now.
You make it fun.
So we ask that
you get well very
soon.
Love,
Tom
Hundley

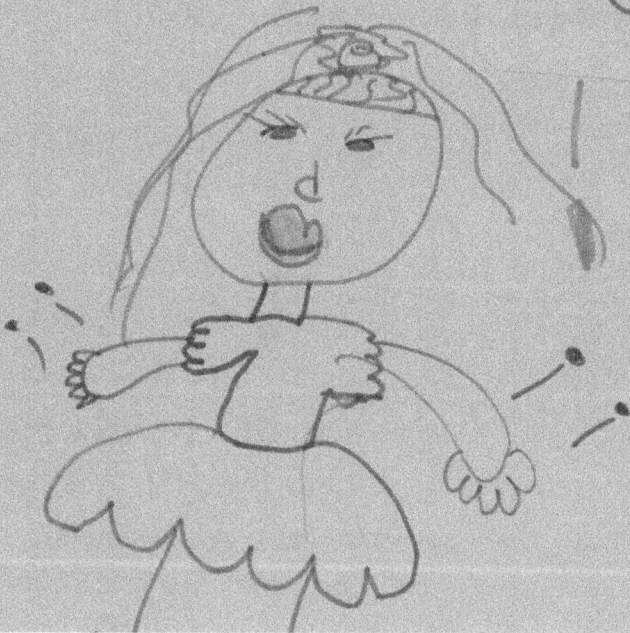

# Chapter 10

## Triple Whammy

☞ . . . the trying of your faith worketh patience. But let patience have her perfect work, that ye may be perfect and entire, wanting nothing.

*James 1: 3-4*

The long corridor leading to the hospital's extensive radiation suite was deceptive. From the top down, the walls on both sides were painted brilliant sky blue. On the left side, fanciful flowers of every variety adorned the lengthy landscaped walkway. On the right, billowing clouds floated freely on the expansive canvas. Painted to depict a walk in the park, the colorful passageway only thinly veiled the valley of the shadow of death.

The first time I entered the corridor, I held Amos's hand and walked the colorful plank with confidence. Walking unaided and medically insured, I thanked God to be alive. I praised the Lord for new mercies daily. While inaccurate Internet information had disappointed me before, and even though the doctors had explained the procedures in detail, I still wasn't quite sure what to expect with these external radiation treatments. For now, it was enough to know God was with me, and His grace was sufficient.

The corridor's vivid colors ended abruptly as Amos and I turned the corner. The passageway opened into a large waiting room with two long rows of padded chairs. We passed a child's play area. A tabletop labyrinth with colorful wooden beads sat atop a child-sized table. At the far end of the room, the receptionist fielded questions from patients waiting in a short line. She wore a colorful and stylish print blouse and smiled warmly as I approached the desk. I too flashed a smile and announced my arrival.

"I'll let them know you're here, Ms. Pace," Beverly responded cheerfully.

I took a seat next to Amos and looked around. This was the place, and these were the faces I'd see every day for five weeks—twenty-five days—of external radiation treatments to the pelvis.

The nurse called me and led the way into an open area with a long counter. An oversized electronic scale flashed my weight in glowing red digits. Next, she ushered me into a small exam room. I sat alone for a while but decided to call for Amos before the radiation oncologist arrived. Like it or not, Amos was invited. We were in this together. Today's session involved marking the pelvic region with permanent tattoos and sizing me for the customized lead shields for use during treatments. The precise field or target for the radiation beam had to be calculated as close to my unique body contour as possible. The reason radiation can be so deadly is that it destroys both the healthy cells along with the malignant ones, just like chemotherapy.

On the first day of treatment, I met a handsome young male radiation technologist with a winning smile. He escorted me to the treatment area. Walking slightly ahead of me, he turned to ask, "Are you nervous?"

"No," I replied, "'cause Jesus is with me."

The young man smiled broadly and nodded like he understood. At this point in my travels, I confessed Christ's presence at every available opportunity. There was no point in anyone being deluded. Just because it *appeared* no one was with me, that didn't mean I walked alone. Moment by moment, I affirmed Christ's presence whether I felt Him or not. Faith in Christ is based on the fact of His Word, not on feelings.

On Monday, March 26, I experienced the first four-hour chemotherapy session. Afterward I trooped dutifully downstairs to prepare for the first radiation treatment. The linear accelerator requires a spacious room to accommodate the immense rotating machine. Stretched prone on the hard surface, a modest drape covered my midsection. It wasn't necessary to undress completely. I simply lowered my slacks and underwear to the knees. The technologist snapped custom-fitted lead shields into the machine's housing and locked it securely. Treatment consisted of four blasts to the pelvic area: to the left and right sides, and then the top and bottom view. All in all, the actual treatment time required less than ten minutes. I felt no particular sensation as the radiation beams struck their intended target. The process was much like getting a regular X-ray. Yet, I knew that unless the Holy Spirit came alongside and protected me from the horrendous side effects of the cumulative toxicity of the daily radiation and the weekly chemotherapy, the flood of poisons in my body would overtake me for sure.

I had a standing date with Amos on Mondays and Fridays. At the beginning of the week, he sat with me in the chemotherapy suite. At week's end, we strolled the colorful corridor before and after radiation exposure. Gracious friends and neighbors chauffeured me on Tuesdays and Wednesdays. Michele, both willing and available, generously offered her services on Thursdays for the duration of treatment. How God provided during these weekday visits with my thoughtful husband and considerate friends. We talked and laughed on the way to the hospital and sometimes stopped for lunch if I wasn't too tired. Dana joined Amos and I during one chemotherapy session. I praised God for my daughter's courage and willingness to come with us.

One friend's unexpected cancellation had me scrambling to find a replacement.

*Who's free to take me to the hospital tomorrow, Lord?*

As evening approached, I called a friend from the Asbury fellowship.

"Are you available to take me to the hospital in the morning?" I asked. "My radiation treatment is at ten and I need a ride to the hospital," I explained.

The next morning Lois arrived around nine o'clock. When I opened the front door, she stumbled into the foyer and hugged me tight.

"I didn't want to come," she confessed. "I've seen people with cancer. So sickly looking and baldheaded. I didn't want to see you like that," she said. "But you look wonderful."

I immediately understood her dilemma. During my work as a volunteer chaplain, I'd seen ravaging physical deterioration in some cancer patients, while others seemed to experience few side effects from treatment. No two patients were alike. Lois and I talked and laughed all the way to the hospital, and praised the Lord for his grace and mercy to us both.

For the next four weeks, I moved through the weekly routine of the Monday chemotherapy session, and then the Monday-through-Friday radiation treatment with as much grace as the Lord allowed. On the weekends, I rested in order to repeat the routine again. The first two weeks went smoothly: I experienced only mild episodes of nausea but never vomited even once. Truly there was nothing wrong with my appetite. I never even felt the need to take more than a couple of Zofran tablets. The pharmacy charged over $700 for this anti-nausea medication.

"No wonder there's no cure," one friend quipped.

I praised the Lord for Amos's insurance coverage requiring only a meager $15 co-payment.

As the weeks progressed, however, the cumulative toxicity of both treatments took their inevitable toll. I experienced a crushing fatigue beyond description, a very common side effect of both chemotherapy and radiation treatment. Bed rest typically cured this malady in an afternoon, but it just kept returning relentlessly, day after tiring day. The real culprit was persistent diarrhea. My sore behind needed rest, and plenty of it. Weak and disheartened, I missed one radiation treatment but dutifully dressed and faced the music the next day.

Out-of-town guests visited during the third week of treatments.

"The retirees have arrived," Susan, my older sister from Denver, exclaimed. I opened the front door wide that Thursday afternoon to welcome her and my dad from Chicago. They had traveled together after connecting in Cincinnati.

"All surgeries are over and everybody's healed," she added enthusiastically.

Unfortunately, Dana was off to Disney World for her high school team's annual robotics competition, so she missed her grandfather, Aunt Susan, and cousin Stephanie, who arrived from Chicago on Saturday. Coming into the home stretch, I knew God was seeing me through, just like He promised. Then, on the fifth and final day of chemotherapy, everything changed dramatically.

As soon as I raised my head to check the glowing red numbers on the digital clock, I knew immediately something wasn't quite right. It was quiet in the house, as usual. Amos slept soundly as I propped myself unsteadily on one elbow. Having shared a bed with him for twenty-six years, I had no intention of disturbing his rest due to restless night travels. No need to create undue alarm. The numbers 4:53 glowed eerily in the darkness. The sensation of vertigo completely distorted the room's familiar shapes and shadows. Squinting now, I sensed the clock moving . . . not the numbers, but the clock itself. The entire ceiling rolled sharply to the left. Next, the corners shifted at a completely distorted angle, then turned again as if on some continuously moving conveyor belt gone haywire.

*This is a bad dream, Irene.*

The unexpected dizzy spell rendered all efforts to keep my eyes open completely futile. I was trapped on some crazy, fun house treadmill, and I couldn't get off. *Close your eyes and wake up from this nightmare!*

To awaken before dawn was certainly nothing new. Since the hysterectomy in late January, frequent predawn bathroom visits disturbed my rest with increasing annoyance. If it wasn't the urge to urinate, then persistent night sweats often left me soaking wet in the middle of the night. But now, dizziness completely surpassed any urgency to urinate. Uncontrolled spinning forced my head back into the soft pillow. Groggy and disoriented, I eased my legs to the side of the bed. Slowly I stood upright, then stumbled toward the bathroom door. The sideways pull of gravity thrust me forcibly into the doorjamb. *Ouch!*

*Grab the sink before you fall,* I barked the mental command to myself. In this muddled state, I extended my hand to reach the sink counter just in time. With one quick turn, I landed less than squarely on the toilet. Praise God the seat was down!

*Lord, just let me make it back to my bed without falling on the floor.*

The ten o'clock appointment loomed overhead like a dark thundercloud. With four hours before show time, I was sure to feel fine . . . just fine, thank God. I groped my way back to bed. Opening my eyes was risky business. I reached for soft comforter fabric to orient myself in the spinning darkness. Squinting briefly, I closed my eyes to maintain equilibrium. The last thing I wanted was to awaken Amos unnecessarily. Crashing headlong into our bed simply would not do. I eased into bed and settled uncomfortably under the covers. Decidedly off balance, my head and limbs hung heavily even on the horizontal plane. A crushing, debilitating fatigue flooded the body and penetrated my soul. Through closed eyes, I mentally searched for whatever rest remained, however fitful. Soon I had to rise and shine and face the music that Monday morning. The fifth and final day of chemotherapy treatment started like a whirlwind roller-coaster ride headed downhill fast.

*It's a good thing there's nothing too hard for God,* I thought before drifting back to sleep in the early-morning haze.

I awakened to the sound of the front door opening and closing and glanced at the clock. The red numerals 6:24 glowed less brightly now. The predawn darkness gave way to morning light, but the dazed and dizzy feeling persisted. Amos must be driving Dana to school for her 6:50 chemistry class, I thought. If he didn't stop for coffee and a bagel, he'd return right after the start of the morning news at seven o'clock. I knew Dana appreciated this Monday-morning ride. Still on cloud nine from the Disney World trip, she was counting days with typical adolescent anticipation before her high school's sophomore cotillion in just two weeks. I didn't have the energy to shop for a formal gown, so Dana's art teacher Lisa stood valiantly in the gap for me, as had so many others while I recuperated.

Whenever Dana and I shopped together, it sometimes took hours of nonstop shopping to find something suitable *and* affordable. Yet, when Dana and Lisa returned with a formal-length dress bag from Lord & Taylor in less than two hours as giddy as schoolgirls, I was dumbfounded. How did they find the perfect dress so quickly? Dana modeled the gown and looked absolutely stunning. Iridescent coral satin shimmered in the afternoon light. The strapless dress with its narrow bodice accentuated her curves. The gathered, scalloped hem looked like something Scarlett O'Hara wore in *Gone with the Wind*. Like a butterfly emerging from the chrysalis, Dana—

a beautiful, confident young woman coming to terms with womanhood and sensuality—fit the prom dress. I could just imagine her elegant entrance. I could hear what passed for music nowadays. I pictured her spinning . . . jumping and bumping on the dance floor.

Shifting the focus to the discomfort of my present reality, I whirled and twirled without the benefit of a disc jockey. The pressing urge to use the bathroom competed with the gravitational pull of the revolving room. I lurched forward, unsteady on bare feet again. Plopping down on the john before I fell, I rocked rhythmically while the room spun completely out of control. Dizziness jettisoned me into total disorientation. I was losing ground fast. I rose slowly from the toilet seat, my spindly legs weak and wobbly. Even before standing, I realized, ruefully, that one glance in the mirror would tell the tale. Caught in a tailspin, I saw through squinting, baggy eyes the reflection of a woman in the throes of a deep descent. I looked positively seasick. My complexion is usually a warm milk chocolate brown, but this morning I was turning slightly green around the gills.

The revolving room deceived me. *I* wasn't really in a tailspin. My *stomach* was the real villain. A wave of nausea, rising and cresting from deep within my belly, crashed into my consciousness with savage fury. I grasped the edges of the sink and bent low to spill my guts into the gaping hole just in the nick of time. How I hated the stench and heaving. The room's relentless orbit dutifully rocked me to the left side. I rinsed my mouth and face with cool water just before the wave crashed again. Fast and furiously, I vomited once more. Thank God I didn't throw up on the floor. Creating extra work infuriated me.

*Do you mean to tell me that this is what I've been missing all these weeks, Lord?*

While I suppressed the urge to laugh out loud, I could not restrain the next bilious heave into the toilet bowl. *This is ridiculous.* I only have one more chemo session to go . . . one more time, and it's all over. After today, there would be no more painful insertion of the IV into my arm. No more taping it securely and carefully positioning my outstretched arm to avoid injury. No more sitting patiently in the reclining chair for 240 minutes watching the steady drip of chemicals—the anti-nausea medication, the Cisplatin, and the diuretics—flow into my veins. No more hobbling repeatedly to the bathroom dragging the IV pole in fervent hope I would not wet my pants. No more! All that mattered now was getting dressed and driving to Philadelphia. After today, no more chemotherapy!

*The waves obey you, Lord. You command the oceans and the waves of nausea too. You proved that during the first week when treatment began, and you calmed any raging seasickness.*

So why am I throwing up now?

*Okay, Father. You're in charge. If today's the day for vomiting, thanks for not allowing this to happen continually for the past four weeks. This is not a pretty picture, but you can handle it. Thank you, Lord Jesus. Please bring Amos home quickly.*

I don't know why, but at that moment, I recalled the first day of chemotherapy treatment when I met Annamma, the chemotherapy nurse. Pleasant and efficient, she ran a tight ship in the spacious, two-person chemotherapy suite on the hospital's sixth floor. Not long after making introductions, formidable and intimidating giants reared their ugly, bald heads.

"You know your hair is going to fall out," she said with matter-of-fact confidence. She seemed to leave no room for anything other than my nodding consent.

"No, it isn't," I replied, calmly matching her air of certainty. She didn't know I had asked my heavenly Father from the start if I could keep my hair. My two oncologists had told me my hair wouldn't fall out. I never went wig shopping with my hairdresser Pearl.

The nurse in the pink smock didn't look convinced at all. Quite naturally, I didn't want any part of chemotherapy treatment. Who would? While these powerful drugs effectively destroy cancer cells, the main drawback is their inability to differentiate between cancerous and healthy tissue. My gynecological oncologist ordered Cisplatin, a potent medication which slows or stops the growth of cancer cells by affecting DNA function. The lethal side effects of this drug make a strong case for the cure being worse than the disease. The long list reads more like a treatment plan gone awry than a time-tested approach to halt the spread of cancer. Using Cisplatin can result in severe nausea and vomiting, temporary hair loss, neuropathy (loss of feeling and/or numbness and tingling in the hands and feet), severe diarrhea, kidney damage, bone marrow suppression, abnormal fatigue, and total hearing loss. In rare cases, seizures can occur. Chemotherapy also can lead to appetite loss. I had already lost fifteen of one hundred thirty pounds during the two weeks following surgery, and I was slowly regaining it back. Any inability to keep my food down would be a disaster. I would look emaciated, suffer malnourishment, and I wouldn't have a thing to wear that fit.

The amiable nurse read me my rights and pointed to the bottom line requiring my signature before the first four-hour treatment could begin. *Help me Jesus,* I prayed silently before scribbling my name illegibly on the standardized form. The faint of heart need not apply.

But now, at home in my bathroom, my heart wasn't the organ giving me trouble. Instead, a deep rumbling in my bowels took center stage. I spun around from facing the toilet in total surrender to the dreaded triple whammy: dizziness, dry heaves, and diarrhea.

*Lord, I know you're here with me. I know it. You've got this 'cause I just can't handle it!*

The internal pressure created havoc and emptied my insides in continuing billows. Flushing the toilet did not eliminate the foul odors mingling in the small room. Exhausted from the exertion and effort to vacate from both ends, my weak head hung limply from bent shoulders.

*Lord, I know you're here. This is impossible. Where is Amos? Send him home on the double, Father.*

By the time I heard the garage door open and close, I lacked the strength to even call Amos's name. On entering our bedroom, I knew Amos expected to find me still in bed.

"Irene," he called. "Today's the last day of chemo. You made it," he added cheerfully.

"Help me, honey. I'm sick," I moaned.

Rushing to my aid, he stopped in his tracks. Was it what he saw or what he smelled? I'm not sure.

"What happened?" he asked blankly.

"I'm dizzy and . . . ," my voice trailed. I reluctantly allowed the wave of nausea and accompanying dry heave to overtake me.

"Get the bucket," I pleaded, knowing I had no strength to stand should I vomit again.

Amos returned with the green bucket. He gently stroked my back as I lowered my face, held on tightly with both hands, and heaved again. After Amos left the bathroom I heard distinctive, touch-tone beeps as he dialed the telephone.

Growing progressively weaker, I closed my eyes to keep the room from spinning into another orbit altogether and taking me with it. I could hear Amos talking as if across a long distance. Several pauses punctuated his conversation then he launched into a short explanation. "She's being treated for cancer," I heard him say.

When he returned to the bathroom door, he looked aggravated. "I left a message with the answering service. The doctor will call back," he announced. "Is there anything I can do?"

"Pray," I responded in earnest.

If anyone could get a prayer through, Amos could. His love for the Lord Jesus Christ, for me, and for his daughters endeared him to me in hundreds of ways. Plenty of water accumulates under the bridge in twenty-six years of marriage, but instead of stagnating, it was a well of water springing up. While Amos's youthful good looks and life-of-the-party disposition made him appear younger than his years, the events of the preceding twelve months had, like chemotherapy and radiation, obviously taken a cumulative toll.

In early January 2000, I was involved in a car accident (praise God no one was seriously injured) that ripped off the front end of his Acura. He flew home from Denver on the next plane smoking to assure himself I was unhurt and check on his car. A few weeks later trouble crashed into Dana's life. Any honest parent will confess that the anger and heavy sullenness of adolescence can erupt without warning at any moment. Over innumerable phone calls back and forth from Denver, Amos's voice registered concern for his youngest daughter's welfare. He returned home again to support Dana and me. We needed help. In March, one month after getting her driver's license, Amos was home the day Lorraine accidentally rammed the rear end of a neighbor's car in my Chevy. Thank God it was only a minor fender bender, but it ended up costing nearly $500 not to involve the insurance company.

On April Fools' Day 2000, Lorraine received her congratulatory letter from Cornell. Unfortunately, Amos's pending layoff in late April overshadowed her good news. After a short business trip to Los Angeles, the pink slip arrived on April 28, only two days before Cornell required a deposit. Very few couples relish a spouse's layoff notice, especially without another job in sight, but Amos was philosophical.

"It was good while it lasted," he said.

Personally and publicly, I rejoiced. *It is finished!* God closed the door on his eighteen-month commute to Denver.

The roofing contractor showed up in May and wanted an additional $900 Amos hadn't figured on to complete the job. Lorraine graduated high school in mid-June. By faith, Amos agreed to plans to rent a tent and host an elaborate garden party for seventy-five guests. Lora and her family catered the affair. Take it from me, it was worth every penny to thoroughly enjoy the party and visit with our guests without any concern for keeping the food hot and the beverages cold. Two days before the party, I mailed a $1,700 payment to Cornell, the first of ten monthly tuition installments. In July, Lockheed Martin offered Amos a systems engineering position. In August Lorraine left for college, and Dana started voice lessons. Frankly, the fall months blurred with activity. I serviced new school clients and observed Dana adjust to "only child" status. Amos was back home, and while he wasn't picky, he appreciated more than the occasional home-cooked meal. In September, he started a fitness regimen and gave me a membership to a nearby gym where I worked out at least four mornings a week after dropping Dana off for school at 6:45. Then, the blood-tinged discharge started the first weekend in November.

What a roller-coaster ride for him! Through diagnosis, surgery, and now these treatments, caring for a sick wife required round-the-clock prayer and attention. Even through squinting eyes, my husband looked exhausted . . . weary, worn, and plum tuckered out.

Bowed in the bathroom, I prayed. I heard Amos praying in the bedroom: *Help her, Holy Ghost. Help my wife.* The storm might be raging, but I believed with certainty and calm assurance our heavenly Father heard us.

The ringing telephone interrupted spiritual communication. The doctor's office instructed Amos to beat a path to the hospital as quickly as possible. In all likelihood, I was severely dehydrated. Only the Holy Ghost could help as I struggled out of the bathroom, bucket in hand. I sat gingerly on the edge of the bed, dropped my head in the bucket, and vomited again.

"You've got to get dressed," said Amos stoically.

"Yeah . . . but I really need to shower first. I don't want to go smelling like this," I responded with a heavy sigh.

Since taking a shower required *standing,* the persistent dizziness rendered a stand-up shower simply out of the question. A quickie sponge bath offered the only option for bodily refreshment now. I held Amos's hand and followed him like a blind woman. Every time I tried to open my eyes, the room spun and whirled in dizzying betrayal. Once inside Dana's bathroom, he helped me undress, then ran some water into the tub. I felt pressure building in my bowel, which forced me to the commode. Amos gently lowered me into the tub and soaped the washcloth. I blindly gave myself a few quick swipes in strategic spots. After a quick rinse, I was done. Amos extended a strong arm to lift me out of the tub. He dried and steadied me, and then led me back into our bedroom. He pulled articles of clothing from my armoire. I dressed and pulled a comb through my hair. Ready to go at last, I mentally prepared for final departure.

"Will you please get the bucket?" I requested, hoping to avoid a crash landing.

If someone could have videotaped footage of me leaving the house, it would be priceless. In one hand, I carried the trusty green bucket close to my body like an indispensable, timeworn blanket. Amos clasped the other. Through the hallway and down the stairs into the foyer, my eyes squinted, and my legs trembled. The kitchen appeared like a desert oasis. I felt an irrepressible urge to plop into one of the wooden chairs. Facing the music is one thing. My contorted face in the bucket was something else again!

*Lord, just help me . . . help me, Jesus.*

As soon as I raised my head from the bucket, I felt the insistent rumbling of yet another loose stool.

"Help me, Amos. I've got to go to the bathroom again. Quick."

I barely made it to the downstairs bathroom before what was left in my lower intestines exploded once again.

At the base of the staircase, I looked up at what appeared to be Mount Everest. "I can make it. I have to make it," I whispered.

*Lord, you've been our help throughout all generations. Don't leave us now!*

With Amos at my side, we mounted the stairs together one step at a time. The open front door, swung wide for easy passage, beckoned me out into the light of day and the start of a critical journey. Squinting momentarily before closing my eyes, I could feel the warmth and see bright sunshine reflecting from the hood of Amos's shiny burgundy Acura. We were out the door.

*We've come this far by faith leaning on the Lord. Hallelujah!*

Amos led me around to the passenger side and opened the car door. I fell heavily into the low seat. The full force of gravity yanked my body to the left and jammed my elbow into the center console. *Oooooww!*

"Get the bucket," I directed weakly, indifferent to space limitations in the front seat. Amos reentered the house. He tossed the bucket in the backseat and handed me some plastic grocery bags. Easing slowly out the driveway, he backed into the street.

Riding with my eyes closed lengthened my perception of time. "Are we there yet," I asked about ten minutes into the forty-minute trip.

"Are you all right?" Amos asked intermittently as he skillfully maneuvered his prized Legend through highway traffic. Dizziness I knew he could handle. The onset of vomiting or a bout of diarrhea would not sit well on his gray leather interior.

The entrance to the hospital at Thirty-fourth and Spruce streets is a classic study in inefficient traffic flow. All too often the congested cross traffic crowding Spruce Street, combined with oncoming traffic on Thirty-fourth Street, rendered a left turn onto Spruce virtually impossible. During four weeks of daily visits for radiation treatment, the valet parking area was sometimes completely inaccessible. Today, as God would have it, traffic was minimal. Amos pulled smoothly into the covered parking zone. He quickly left the car, barely waiting for the attendant to hand him a parking ticket.

"I'll get you a wheelchair," he assured me.

Normally there are at least five or six wheelchairs at the curbside entrance, but not today. Weak and woozy, I could not move without help. Barely able to open my eyes, I squinted long enough to see the parking attendant motion for me to get out of the car. Clearly he didn't understand. Straining to discover Amos's whereabouts, I could hardly keep my eyes open without reeling to the left. The nauseous feeling threatened menacingly.

*Not now, Lord. Please not now.*

"I'm going to help you, Irene. There are no wheelchairs in sight . . . not even in the lobby," Amos announced with regret.

"Go figure," I murmured. "Get the plastic bag."

Once inside the hospital lobby, Amos led me to a chair and went off in search of an elusive wheelchair. I needed some wheels to make it upstairs. Unfortunately, he had taken the plastic bag. Let's hope he didn't have to carry me.

*Lord, please don't let me throw up all over myself in this hospital lobby. Help me, Lord Jesus. Help me to "keepittogether."*

After what seemed like an eternity, Amos returned triumphant. I eased into the rolling chair and held the plastic bag in my lap. I waited only briefly for the nursing assistant to call my name. After explaining the morning's events, the blood pressure check told the whole story. At 70/40 my blood had turned to sludge. I would be admitted to the hospital just as soon as a bed became available. The Rx: start an IV immediately to counteract dehydration.

Now the very nature of time seemed to change. We waited only about twenty short minutes for a room. A smiling attendant placed me carefully on a gurney and wheeled me to the fourth floor with Amos at my side. I only opened my eyes momentarily as the elevator door parted at the fourth floor. The impressionist painting on the wall seemed vaguely familiar. The fourth floor . . . the same floor I lived on for seven days following the hysterectomy in January. Today was March 23, 2001 . . . exactly three months to the day of the surgery. In a matter of minutes, the white-coated nurse deftly started the IV. It was the same nurse who compassionately handled my discharge procedures on January 29. I had given her a colorful bouquet from the many thoughtful floral gifts I had received during my hospital stay. Now she too remembered me.

"I thought I recognized your name on the chart, Ms. Pace. What are you doing here?" Before I could answer, she leaned closer with only one question on her mind: "Is that your hair?" she blurted out incredulously, her eyes wide with curiosity.

I smiled faintly. Tugging repeatedly on a generous handful of hair from the right side of my scalp was an unexpected blessing. *Isn't God good!*

# Part III

**Survival and Triumph**

# Chapter 11

## Do You Know How Hard This Is?

☙ Thou therefore endure hardness, as a good soldier of
Jesus Christ.

*II Timothy 2:3*

Monday's euphoria of not having to undergo the fifth and
final chemotherapy treatment quickly faded Friday morning when
I expected to end five weeks of radiation treatments. The chief
resident delivered the bad news. She informed me *twenty-seven*
courses of radiation completed the treatment protocol, *not twenty-
five,* as I so eagerly anticipated. Dr. Eleanor Harris, my radiation
oncologist, was away for a conference and would not return until
Monday.

"She said five weeks, and it's been five weeks," I complained
impatiently. "I've only missed two treatments, and no one told me
I had to make them up," I protested, verbalizing my utter
disappointment at the prospect of returning two more times. Here
I thought I had crossed the finish line, only to discover I was short
by two steps. I didn't want to run this leg of the marathon race
any longer, and I wasn't afraid to say so. "I'm through with this.
Check with Dr. Harris. It's over," I declared.

The dark-haired doctor urged me to complete the full twenty-
seven-day course of radiation.

"It's important to receive the full dosage now," she said. "If
you stop short of the full course, it's not like you can go back for

two more treatments if there is recurrence. It's like insurance," the chief resident explained. "Besides, you've come this far without any major complications from the chemo or the radiation. What are two more treatments?" she appealed.

*How can she ask me that so glibly, Lord?*

After all I'd been through, the mention of recurrence stopped me dead in my disappointed tracks. Yet, at that moment, two additional treatments seemed like a barefoot trek to the moon and back. I didn't want any more radiation, but I didn't want to be foolhardy either, especially after coming this far.

"Check with Dr. Harris and have her call me over the weekend," I relented. At least I could buy some time. "I'm not happy about coming back for two more treatments, but I want to do what's best."

I absolutely refused to dwell on the possibility of cancer's recurrence. Once, while sitting in the waiting room for my date with the linear accelerator, I flipped through *Survivor*, a magazine aimed at cancer patients and their families. The magazine featured a man the editors named "Cancer Survivor of the Year." I perused the piece with more than a passing interest. This man had experienced multiple recurrences over a number of years in different areas of his body. The writer applauded his courageous battle against this deadly legion of diseases. I slowly closed the magazine's pages. I couldn't finish reading. At that moment, any thought of recurrence was just too heavy.

**My yoke is easy and my burden is light, Irene.**

*Thank you, heavenly Father. I hear you. In the name of Jesus, I say thank you. I don't have to think about that now,* I recalled as I sat rigidly on the exam table. The chief resident promised to contact the radiation oncologist and have her call me.

After the full twenty-seven-day course of radiation treatments finally ended, I gladly rested my sore behind. I'd grown progressively weak over the past six weeks. The cumulative toxicity of both the chemotherapy and the radiation treatments took a devastating toll, both physically and emotionally. While I did not experience any hair loss or appetite suppression, the effects of the constant diarrhea were downright depressing. Nonetheless, I knew I must gird my loins for the third and final phase of treatment: internal high-dosage radiation (HDR).

The clinical description of HDR to the vagina sent cold chills down my spine. Internal radiation, also called brachytherapy, places the source of high-energy rays inside the body, as close to the cancer cells as possible. Although I'd had the hysterectomy, chemotherapy, and external radiation, the aggressive curative approach to cervical cancer is not for the squeamish. The goal of internal radiation is to eliminate any remaining cancer cells that the combination of chemotherapy and external radiation had not killed. Unlike external radiation treatment, HDR delivers very intense radiation to a small area of the body and limits the dose to normal tissues. The gynecological oncologist and the radiation oncologist concurred. Both prescribed internal HDR to the vagina to destroy any remaining cancer cells at the vulnerable vaginal cuff. The cervix is the lower, tapered part of the pear-shaped uterus leading into the top of the vagina. Both specialists identified the vaginal cuff, the internal area at the top of the vagina, as a fragile site where cancer can recur.

Once a week for three weeks, a hollow canister would be placed inside my vagina, and a radioactive substance—radium, cesium, iodine, or phosphorus—would be injected through a lead tube inserted into the vagina. The first of the three sessions would take about ninety minutes to complete the required setup procedures. During this time, the radiation oncologist and a physicist would make precise calculations for the amount of time the radioactive source would remain inside me. I would also need a barium injection to highlight the lower intestines during the procedure.

Prior to starting internal radiation treatments, I simply refused to worry about it beforehand. I decided to handle internal radiation in the same way I thought about injecting myself with Procrit or sitting through four hours of chemotherapy.

"I'll just cross that bridge when I come to it," I said resolutely.

*You've brought me this far by faith, Father God. I've come too far to turn back now. You'll get me through this. I know you will. This is the fire, and you said I wouldn't get burned. The waters and the floods didn't overtake me, Lord. Just like you promised. So I believe you, Father. I'm not even going to smell like smoke. I trust you, Lord.*

About a week before the internal treatments began, I had a scheduled follow-up appointment with my surgeon, the gynecological oncologist. I mentioned experiencing some neuropathy, a feeling of numbness in my feet. She checked the abdominal incision and planned to conduct yet another pelvic exam. Straddled spread eagle with my feet in the stirrups, I was totally unprepared for what happened next as her gloved fingers touched the outer labia.

"Ohhhhhhhhwwww," she muffled a gasp. "I cannot . . . you're too raw and irritated . . . it's too red. I don't want to hurt you by putting in a speculum," she stated somberly.

With a determined look in her steel blue eyes, the doctor motioned for her assistant to help me out of the stirrups. I slid back on the narrow table and struggled against gravity and my gravest fears.

*Lord Jesus, what is she saying? I'm supposed to start the first internal treatment next week, Father. What is she saying, Lord?*

"Do you know how hard this is?" I implored, struggling to control my mind and voice. She touched my arm.

*Does she know what it feels like to hear her words and see her reaction to the sight of my once-delicate vagina, Lord? Does she know how hard this is?*

"I'm scheduled for internal radiation next week," I explained, fighting desperately for the composure not to burst into tears. I bit my lip and hoped against hope for a reprieve. "Can I postpone that until I heal?" I asked, my voice rising.

*Does she know how hard this is, Lord?*

"You do need to go for that," she gently urged, squashing my hopes. "The rawness and swelling from the radiation will eventually subside," she offered.

Usually I could joke with this specialist about *something*. To me, a lighthearted approach *always* helped. It proved a rock-solid commitment to believe God's command to be of good cheer . . . not to be discouraged or dismayed. I was determined to find *some* light in the midst of the darkness . . . even a flicker of hope against the dreary, burdensome shroud of cancer treatment. Yet today, while I searched diligently, the elusive needle in the cancer treatment haystack totally eluded me. Her reassuring words offered very little comfort. Precipitously close to losing hope, I was unable to encourage myself, but I could pray.

*This is impossible, Lord Jesus.*

"I have not been through this myself. I only see it through the eyes of my patients," she began. "Yes, I know it's hard, but it's in patients like yourself that I see the strength and courage to go on," she said. "Get dressed, and we'll talk."

*I'm talked out, Lord. There's nothing left.*

After the surgeon and her assistant left the room, I sat silently on the table's edge, momentarily unable to move.

*You said this flood wouldn't overtake me, Lord. You promised.*

Easing slowly, deliberately from the table's edge, I fought back hot tears while I dressed and tied my tennis shoes.

*I'm on the edge, Lord. On the very edge. If you don't fight for me, there's no way I'm going to win. Only with you, Lord, are all things possible.*

During the five weeks and two days of radiation treatments, I had often noticed the half-open door to the internal radiation suite. As I walked through the long corridor to the waiting room reserved for external radiation patients, I shoved the thought of HDR out of my mind. Now it was time to enter these anterooms as well. It wasn't that the radiation oncologist and her chief resident had not explained the procedure and answered my questions. It was just extremely difficult to concentrate on the physical and emotional realities of what would happen next.

"The first treatment takes the longest," Dr. Harris explained on the first day of HDR.

I had read the American Cancer Society booklets, called their hotline, and surfed the Internet. Beyond that, I didn't know how I'd react. I only briefly entertained the notion of joining a cervical cancer support group. I had taken the initiative to speak privately with the social worker on staff in HUP's radiation department, but in my mind, I just wasn't ready for group discussion. Once again, my best bet involved simply showing up for treatment.

The nursing staff made every conceivable effort to provide some comfort on the treatment table, but this was definitely not a comfortable place. Much larger than the room where the doctor yanked the catheter from my bladder, I lay on the table and stared at the ceiling at least twelve feet above my head. The room's dimensions accommodated an immense machine to my far right. The coldness served medical technology. It did not pretend to meet my needs. From my vantage point on the table, I could see through a large glass window into an adjacent room where a bank of computers completely lined one wall. When the nurse returned to check me after I donned the required hospital gown, I asked for a blanket.

The first treatment required about ninety minutes because the physicist needed to calculate the precise dosage of the radioactive isotope to be used. Actual radiation exposure to the vagina would not exceed ten minutes. The prep took the bulk of the time. In contrast, the next two sessions normally only required about ten to fifteen minutes in total, since the required calculations were already completed.

*It doesn't matter how long it takes, Lord. Just help them get it right.*

Before radiation could begin, it was necessary to illuminate the internal field with a barium solution injected into my rectum through a slender tube. Lying on a metal pan on the exam table with my knees up, a crushing heaviness began to overwhelm me. Two doctors and a nurse attended during the prepping process. First, Dr. Harris inserted the hollow canister. Next her chief resident, the woman who had urged me to undergo the two additional days of external radiation, inserted the tube for the barium highlight into my rectum.

**I'm with you, Irene. I'm always with you.**

*I hear you, Lord. I hear you. Thank you, Lord Jesus. I need you.*

The medical team advised me of the procedure. They would leave the room to check my bowel function on computer screens in the room with the glass window before the actual radiation treatment began. A kind voice mentioned the treatment room was equipped with an intercom. I could call out if I needed anything.

*Help, Lord. Help me to be still and know that I AM God. I need that God right now.*

Shortly afterward, the medical professionals returned. The face of the radiation oncologist clearly registered a look of consternation.

"We need to reinsert the barium tubing," Dr. Harris said. The probe had slipped from my rectum. I lay drenched in a pool of barium solution.

*You've got this, Lord. I know you're with me.*

"Is it going to burn my skin?" I asked, now fully aware of the wet sensation on my bare bottom and the soaking gown clinging to my skin.

"No," she replied. "It's just a little messy for you." A nurse wiped my bottom with some towels and blotted excess liquid from the pan.

*I will trust you, Lord. No matter what, I trust you.*

From the outset, I didn't have much to say. I just kept praying the entire time. Before the procedure began, one of the nurses who knew me from external radiation treatments came in to check on me.

"You're awful quiet today, Ms. Pace. Are you okay?" she remarked.

"Yeah," I acknowledged through prayers that never ceased.

When the radiation oncologist first inserted the canister into my vagina, I inhaled and exhaled slowly, praying with every breath. This was no time to tense up. God was with me moment by moment through this. His promised presence was wonderfully apparent to me this second time, because as the doctors were leaving the room, I started to sing to Him.

"Remember if you need anything, we can hear you," the nurse reminded.

*Victory in Jesus. Victory in Jesus. I have the victory. Victory in Jesus. Satan has got to flee.* It might look like I was lying silently on the exam table, but *in the Spirit,* I was singing the jailhouse rock, just like Paul and Silas in a Bible story recorded in the book of Acts, chapter 16, verse 25.

"Did you say something, Ms. Pace?" asked a voice over the intercom.

"I'm just singing," I replied, surprised someone had heard me.

*Tell me who can stand before me, when I call on that great name. Jesus, Jesus, precious Jesus. I have the victory!*

After the barium tube was reinserted, all was ready, and *in the Spirit,* all was well.

"We're ready to start now," declared the intercom voice.

I heard intermittent clicking like a Geiger counter as the powerful radiation traveled through the lead tubing to its internal target. It didn't hurt, and I didn't focus on its potential to harm me.

**The fire will not burn you, Irene.**

"I have the victory," I sang softly.

From my experience with bowel prep for the CT scan and for surgery, I knew ten minutes was a very short time, so I kept on singing. When it was over, the physicist entered the room with a Geiger counter to insure there was no radiation leakage.

"Everything is fine," he said with a heavy Indian accent.

*Victory in Jesus is much better than fine,* I thought.

Three medical professionals returned to the treatment room. Dr. Harris removed the canister and the barium tubing and helped me sit upright. Wet from the barium spill, I was one step closer to the end of this long, hard journey. With one treatment down, and two to go, the end was in sight.

The following week, I knew what to expect, and I didn't need the barium injection. The third and final internal treatment required only about five minutes. The radiation department had just received a fresh radioactive source. What timing!

*God, you are truly a merciful Father. Thank you. Thank you. Thank you.*

I walked out of the radiation suite for the last time, waving to friends I'd made and hugging others. Finished now, finally finished, Amos and I prepared to leave the hospital.

"Can we stop in the chapel?" I asked.

"Sure," he replied.

I needed to return to this special place one more time. This was where God had met me so many times and heard my prayers, both as a volunteer chaplain and as a patient undergoing treatment. Bending our knees on the padded rest, Amos and I held hands. I silently offered the sacrifice of praise and thanksgiving. I raised my free hand to the hills from where my help had come. What a mighty God we serve!

*You brought me through, Lord. I'm through. Thank you, Jesus. I'm through!*

⊰⊱

Six weeks later, I returned to the radiation oncologist's office. Dr. Harris conducted a pelvic exam and handed me a vaginal dilator to stretch the vaginal walls and keep them supple. The solid plastic cylinder was round on one end and flat on the other. It measured about six inches long and one inch in diameter. After radiation to the pelvis, doctors recommend using a dilator to prevent the formation of scar tissue, which can permanently close the vagina. Although it was not anatomically correct, the cold, hard white stick served an important purpose for the time being. All I needed now was the courage to overcome the psychological hurdle of using it.

The only alternative to using the dilator is to have sexual intercourse several times a week. Now that's an alternative I could get excited about. Unfortunately, my love life wasn't even on the ground floor of resumption. Instead, I wandered aimlessly . . . somewhere in sexual intimacy's subbasement. I wasn't the least bit interested in sex following the six-week checkup. The hysterectomy jettisoned me into instant menopause, and my libido hadn't recovered. The thought of sexual intercourse was just too painful, both physically and emotionally.

"Don't read the instructions first," advised Leslie, one of the nurses in the radiation department. "When you first start to use it, give yourself some privacy and relax," she suggested.

"What about sexual intercourse?" I ventured hesitantly.

I first raised questions about the resumption of intimate sexual relations with my two oncologists who were also gynecologists. They both agreed that medically and physically, the necessary healing had occurred for intercourse to resume. It's what they weren't saying that had me squirrelly: clearly, my emotional and psychological wounds needed more time to heal.

"Go out for a romantic date and have some wine to relax. You'll be fine," Leslie assured.

The first part of her suggestion definitely made sense. How I needed romancing, but I didn't drink alcoholic beverages. Little did I know the vaginal dilator could make me change my mind!

I found it incredibly difficult to use the dilator. At a deep emotional and psychological level, I couldn't bring myself to insert it. My psyche and the remaining vestiges of my sexual identity were far more sensitive than my vagina. I didn't want to do it, I tell you. But I didn't want my vagina to close either. The rock and the hard place seemed like a permanent address.

My maiden voyage using the dilator was more like discovering virgin territory. Tense and tight, I knew without any reservation that if God didn't help me with this, it could not be done. It was absolutely impossible. The first try lasted less than three minutes. Flat on my back, my knees shook uncontrollably. I had barely inserted the dilator halfway inside.

*You've brought me so far, Lord. I still need you.*

I cried a river in the shower that day. I couldn't think about touching that thing with a ten-foot pole for another whole week. *Maybe if it was brown instead of white,* I mused.

*Help, Lord. Help!*

Little by little, I relaxed more and inserted the dilator further inside. But I still could not shake the private agony every time I used it. When I finally read the instructions, I was so glad I waited. While the understanding nurse advised using it three times a week with allowance for sexual intercourse in between, the instructions clearly recommended *daily* use. The sobering finality of the third paragraph stopped me cold: since scarring in the pelvis after radiation can develop over many years, you should continue this schedule for the rest of your life.

*Help me, Jesus! Jesus. HELP!*

Over the next several months, I used the dilator only sporadically. Awkward lovemaking attempts were even less frequent. Amos and I passed like ships in the night on differing courses. Physically stronger now, I exercised regularly and joined a four-week fitness class in the beginning of July. In August, the entire family vacationed in Southern California as Charlotte's guests at her spacious home in Los Angeles. I met Dr. Lyra Gillette, Charlotte's gynecologist friend and now mine, who had helped me with so many gynecological and cancer-related questions before and after treatment. We also drove to San Diego, visited our old neighborhood, and dined with Jacqué, a friend for nearly 20 years, in the open-air ambiance of Horton Plaza, the city's downtown gaslight district.

The next day, we laughed and talked with a very special couple during an unforgettable day at the San Diego Zoo where I fainted while waiting to board the tour bus. We first met back in 1988 when we lived in San Diego. We each became first-time, grateful parents of bouncing baby girls within days of each other back in March 1982. Our beautiful daughters, now mature college women, hadn't been photographed together since they were eighteen months old!

On the morning of September 11, I watched the morning news while I drank a protein drink and straightened the kitchen. I turned off the television at 8:45 and went upstairs to finish preparations for a 9:30 Jazzercise class my neighbor Cecilia conducts. I needed to gather my gear and make one business phone call, so I'd be ready to leave shortly after nine o'clock. My friend Michele signed up for the class too. Today, her husband Bruce had dropped her off at the community center. I planned to drive her home after class.

Entering fully and jubilantly into the spirit of the dance, I cried, "Weeeeeee," when we did the airplane twirls. I loved that move: it made me feel free like a butterfly in flight. Pumping and jumping with the best of them, I did not have the slightest clue to the awful and terrible tragedy unfolding in the unfriendly skies. After class, one woman remarked, "Did you hear? A plane hit the World Trade Center."

"What? No, I didn't hear," I replied, thinking only fleetingly about this "accident" as my heart rate returned to normal.

It wasn't until I drove Michele home from the one-hour class and entered her kitchen that we discovered the horrible news. Bruce directed our attention to unimaginable images on the television set.

"Two planes hit the World Trade Center Towers. Both towers have collapsed," he exclaimed. "You have to see this. It's unbelievable. I know they will show it again," he predicted with accuracy.

Riveted on the television screen, I fell to my knees and raised both hands to heaven.

*LORD, God Almighty. I know you are sovereign. You control ALL things. You reign, Lord. All power is in your hand. Help the people, Lord. Heaven help us all.*

Like many travelers worldwide, I was hesitant about flying after September 11. But deep down, I knew it was only a matter of time before I boarded an airplane again. I flew to Chicago in October. Sue traveled from Denver for our mini-reunion in the Windy City. Afterward I returned to her comfortable home to inhale some Rocky Mountain air for a few days. Two weeks before Christmas 2001, I flew to Chicago again to wrap up some family affairs. My dad had business to conduct in the Sears Tower. Anxious-looking guards manned the electronic arches and conveyor belts at the towering skyscraper's security checkpoints. Dad emptied loose change and his wallet into a small basket. I placed my handbag on the moving conveyor belt. A guard passed the wand around Dad who set off the alarm when he passed through the arch. He forgot to remove his keys.

*This is the price we must pay for our freedom, Lord. Tomorrow isn't promised. And neither is the next moment!*

With God's help, I had come to know with certainty that *now* is a very good time. *Now* is the time to love and laugh, to forgive and forget. Laugh *now* and live life *now*, I'd tell anyone within earshot. Life is a precious, priceless, matchless gift from God. All of it! Every day of it . . . Sick or well, rain or shine, dark or light. Praise God I learned this before 9/11. It's no secret life can mow you down, if you let it. Yet, life remains sacred. In the process of cancer treatment and recovery, I discovered life is definitely worth living . . . even with the challenge of using the dilator even every other day. The Lord willing, I faced the prospect of visiting the oncologist every three months for the next five years to monitor my health status. The Lord willing, I anticipated holidays, graduations, parties, and the joys of everyday, moment-by-moment living. All things considered, I rejoiced wholeheartedly: *life is good!*

I had a "no problem" Pap test and CT scan of the pelvis in early October 2001. At Thanksgiving I praised God for His continuing mercy and favor. And two weeks before Christmas, fully one year to the day of hearing "you have cancer," I emailed my buddies from Chicago.

*The Lord willing, I return to New Jersey tomorrow. I suspect there will be times of flying through clouds, thick gray-white masses that obstruct all vision. I appreciate the spiritual parallel: very often we just cannot see where we are going. We have no clue to the Shepherd's leading. Nevertheless, the faith that pleases God requires that we go out not knowing but trusting the Word of life to light our path, give us hope, and make us free. By God's grace I am free today. Not just free of cancer, but also free from the fear, despair, or anxiety commonly associated with cancer treatment and its aftermath. More importantly, I am free to unfold, to create, and to rejoice. I remain deeply grateful for the joy of your friendship and for your fervent prayers on my behalf. Continued blessings!*

# Chapter 12

## Weeping May Endure, but Joy Comes

> ✠ Then was our mouth filled with laughter, and our tongue with singing . . . They that sow in tears shall reap in joy.

*Psalm 126:2,5*

After a truly joyous Christmas 2001, Amos and I celebrated our twenty-seventh wedding anniversary in style: an on-the-town weekend stay in Philadelphia at the Wyndham Plaza Hotel. From our room on the twenty-fifth floor, the view of the art museum and the plaza below reminded us of grand vistas from Chicago's John Hancock Building before we wed. But more than ever before, my focus remained fixed in the present moment and its joys. The first night we listened to the blues and ate greens and fried catfish at Warm Daddy's near Penn's Landing. We celebrated our anniversary at Don Shula's Steak House. Amos ordered prime rib. I selected succulent seafood. We continued the party with dessert at Zanzibar Blue, Philadelphia's premier jazz club. Thank God for the best seat in the house despite the crowd! We tapped and swayed to the mellow sound of the evening's headliner, a popular jazz saxophonist. The emcee was a personal friend whose smooth voice heralded our private milestone with public congratulations. The next day, we shopped for after-Christmas bargains in Center City, then traveled about forty-five minutes south up I-95 to Longwood Gardens, the renowned 1,050-acre horticultural extravaganza created by wealthy industrialist Pierre S. du Pont. A million holiday lights dazzled visitors of all ages who gaped in awe at the brilliant night sky, despite plummeting temperatures and gusty winds.

After the celebrations ended, I settled into the ebb and flow of a brand new year and continued writing. In March 2002, I returned to Chicago. Sue planned to arrive from Denver within minutes of my flight so dad could pick us up together at O'Hare International Airport. I wrote with regularity now. Two things topped my agenda this trip: lending support to an aging aunt whose husband lay comatose in a hospital on the far South Side and concluding personal family business initiated in December. I was out of town for a week.

The Sunday morning after I returned from Chicago, I was giddy with gratitude: God spared my aunt from lapsing into a diabetic coma. Although I wasn't completely rested, I felt a genuine, heartfelt desire to worship God, to praise and thank Him for yet another deliverance. Sunday worship services started at eight o'clock, and it was important to attend. I wanted to praise the Lord Jesus with praying friends at Asbury United Methodist Church once more. Airplane safety after the tragic events of 9/11 was another reason to rise and praise the Lord. While I always looked forward to returning to the Windy City, air travel is just more stressful now. This was my third trip to Chicago in five months. I was happy to be safe at home. Tired or not, I refused to take my remaining time on earth for granted. God didn't have to keep sending blessings my way. Yet, the soft pillow attracted my head like a magnet.

My thoughts drifted to my elderly aunt. When Sue and I arrived to find her front door ajar, we should have known something was wrong. Asleep on the sofa with the telephone in her hand, we didn't realize her diabetes was to blame. We cooked fish in the unfamiliar kitchen and tried to serve her, but we just couldn't keep her head out of the plate.

Sue held her shoulders while I reached for the telephone. In one instant, looking down at the illuminated numbers on the dial and looking up at the scene with Sue holding my aunt in a dazed stupor, I suffered momentary paralysis.

Sue analyzed my dilemma immediately. From years of experience as an airline employee, she remained calm in this emergency situation.

"It's 9-1-1," she slowly intoned in the calmest, most methodical voice I had ever heard her use.

I snapped out of my stupor and dialed. Sue kept our aunt upright while I made a clean sweep of papers and money scattered across the dining room table. In less than ten minutes, a roomful of paramedics and concerned neighbors came to our rescue. The paramedics measured her blood sugar at thirty. She was fading fast.

"Do you have any juice?" one of the guys asked. "You're going to make something your mother would never let you drink."

He followed me into the kitchen and asked for honey and sugar. I poured cranberry juice into a tall glass and added two heaping spoonfuls each of both sweeteners. My aunt needed to drink this syrupy concoction in a few gulps to quickly elevate her blood sugar level. It was a harrowing twenty minutes as she slowly returned to consciousness and coherency. I shudder to think what would have happened had we hesitated to call 911. My uncle who loved model trains lay comatose in a South Side hospital. The prognosis wasn't good. If the nieces could provide even a little comfort to our aunt, his wife of fifty-seven years, the primary purpose for this visit would be well served.

Despite the emotional energy expended with my aunt, and the draining drama at my uncle's bedside, I treasured the time with the McCullough family. This weeklong visit was especially remarkable because Sue and I shared dad's upstairs attic bedroom. We hadn't shared a bedroom in over forty years. I can't say it was like old times. It was new and fun, much better than the argumentative days when I begged to wear her clothes. I thank God for Susan. Retired now after thirty-three years with Delta Airlines, she's a very special lady. Quite naturally, our long talks well into the night and our early-morning teatime left little room for any privacy to use the vaginal dilator even once while I was away. Now, lying in bed with Amos, his rhythmic breathing clearly signaled lovemaking was not in my immediate future. As he slept peacefully, I slipped quietly out of bed, washed the dilator carefully, returned to my bedside, and prepared to insert it. *He'll never wake up,* I thought.

I sat on the edge of the bed, applying lubricating gel to the thing. The weight of hopeless resignation to the long-term consequences of cervical cancer crushed me. I recoiled at the effects of radiation to my delicate vagina.

Almost everything within me rejected the dehumanizing insertion of this plastic stick. Everything except this: failure to use it and keep my vagina open meant no more sexual intercourse. While sexual gratification and lovemaking do not always involve intercourse, I wasn't focusing on that, for the moment. Besides, my two oncologists had warned that if my vagina closed, not only would it preclude sexual intercourse. It would become impossible to insert a speculum for future internal examination. Stuck between a rock and a hard place, I sighed deeply. If I wanted to keep my vagina open, I had two choices: either enjoy the warmth and intimacy of sexual intercourse with Amos, or insert the cold plastic dilator on a regular basis for ten minutes. From the sound of Amos's breathing, this was a "Plan B" morning. Maybe later this afternoon, we could leisurely make love, but it definitely wasn't going to happen right now.

Just sitting on the bed, my thoughts returned to vignettes of the latest Chicago trip. I pictured my aging aunt, now in her eighties. With my uncle in a coma, she too faced the imminent loss of future intimacy of any kind with the man she loved.

*Life's difficulties just keep crashing in on us, Father.*

Listening to Amos's breathing, I felt so sad. Over the years of our long marriage, there had been some dry spells, but for the most part, we made time for sexual intimacy and gave sexual intercourse high priority. Now, too much heavy baggage cluttered thoughts about my own sexuality and diminishing sexual desire: Was I still attractive to my husband? Could I ever relax enough to enjoy sex again? What if sex was just too painful now? Was it even worth it to keep trying? I looked for some joy, but found trouble and sorrow.

*Just lay back, use this dilator, and get it over with,* I reasoned. I needed to quell the nagging suspicion that sexual satisfaction was forever beyond my grasp. Despite what the books or the Internet reported, perhaps sexual pleasure was a thing of the past, after all. Instinctively, I knew this line of thinking was detrimental. Mentally shaking loose these cobwebs, I encouraged myself: *Come on, Irene. Keep an open mind. That's the only way to avoid a closed vagina.*

*Help me with this, dear Lord. Help me. There's nothing too hard for you, Father.*

Just sitting, holding the lubricated dilator in my hand, I was about to lie back quietly when Amos stirred from sleep. Startled, he sat up on one elbow. He looked puzzled.

"Are you all right? What are you doing?" he asked with seeming alertness. I looked at him but did not reply.

He swung the comforter from across his legs and sat up on his side of the bed.

"Just hold on now. I've got something for you. Grease me up," he offered before rising to use the bathroom. His arrogant tone and the haughty suggestion cut like a scalpel. His attitude severed a raw and sensitive nerve.

I sat on the bedside and blinked repeatedly in stunned silence. *He didn't say that,* I thought. *No. I don't believe he said that. Did you hear that, Lord? Father, help me with this. Help me.*

Amos returned from the bathroom and slipped into bed. With my back to him now and the dilator in my hand, I had a clear choice. I could either make love or use the dilator. It was that simple. I could choose.

*Help me, Lord Jesus.*

Taking a slow, deep breath, I lay back on the bed in silence. Moving into position with my knees bent and legs spread apart, I inserted the dilator and turned my head away. A heavy, unbearable silence filled our room. But the weight of the silence was no match for the hot, heavy tears quietly filling the corners of my eyes. With stinging tears trickling down the sides of my face, I counted time.

*Ten minutes, Lord. Just ten lousy minutes.*

I rose without a word. Once inside the bathroom, I looked in the mirror at my contorted, tear-stained face. The tears, hotter and heavier, came easier now that I had some privacy. My body shook with gut-wrenching sobs.

*Lord, Lord.*

This flood broke the dam.

*I will not, I cannot swallow these tears. It's too much, Lord.*

Waves of sorrow and sadness crashed over me. The weight of grief and anguish broke my heart.

I wiped my eyes and peered into the mirror again. *Who are you, Irene? What has happened to you? This isn't about Amos; it's about you,* I argued.

*What's happening, Father? Have twenty-seven years of marriage come to this? Please help me, Lord.*

I reentered the bedroom to find Amos where I left him. For physical support, I leaned my elbow on the tall armoire. Struggling for composure, I needed to speak, to find my voice in the aftermath of cervical cancer's cruel, long-term consequences and my husband's short-term memory lapse regarding my very vulnerable psyche on this issue. *Have I been with you this long and you still don't know the woman you married,* I mused. The words of a bumper sticker rang true: Speak your mind even if your voice shakes.

*Give me the words to say, Holy Spirit. I need the mind of Christ on this one.*

"You have to understand something, Amos. Just because I had cancer, that doesn't mean I don't have feelings."

I inhaled and stood slightly straighter. The bumper sticker was right: even if your voice shakes.

"Grease me up. That was *so* insensitive," I choked on the uncaring word but continued bravely nonetheless. "It's hard to believe you would be so insensitive to me about this after all I've been through. I know you're affected too, but we have to work this out together, or we're not going to make it." I was gaining momentum. "I've done it plenty of times before, but I'm not going to swallow these tears. Not now and not ever again. If you don't want to make love to me, so be it. But understand this. I have worth and value. I'm somebody special, whether you appreciate me or not." There, I said it.

Standing on God's promise, I returned to the bathroom. The mirror reflected bloodshot, swollen eyes. I didn't look any different than I had a few minutes earlier, but I found my voice. I blew my nose and rinsed my face with several cold splashes. Slightly refreshed, I found my voice.

*Thank you, Lord. Thank you, Father.*

"Irene. Telephone."

Amos's muffled voice faintly registered over the sound of the running water.

*Who could be calling this early on a Sunday morning,* I wondered? I didn't even hear the phone ring. *I can't talk now.*

With the bathroom door closed, I heard Amos's muffled voice mixed with laughter.

Temporarily distracted, I blew my nose.

*Who's he talking to at a time like this? How can he laugh when he knows I'm hurting?*

"Irene. It's for you."

I didn't want to open the door. Not now.

A moment ago, I found my voice. Now, I could barely manage the words, "I can't talk right now."

Sometimes the telephone rings at the most inopportune times. This lifelong friend was among the very first I notified about the diagnosis back in December 2000. Ordinarily, her call merited my immediate attention, no matter what.

*But not today.*

"She needs to talk to you," Amos urged.

I toyed with the idea of barricading the door. Finally, I relented.

I held the cordless phone to my ear with great reluctance. I weakly muttered her name.

"Hey, girl. How ya doing?" she said with exuberant cheerfulness. "I've just got to tell you something hysterically funny."

Under normal circumstances, I loved to hear this woman's latest antics. I often wondered if she missed her calling as a stand-up comedienne. In person, with her wild gestures, impersonations, and facial expressions, she is positively insane. On the phone, her certifiably craziness is equally capable of splitting my sides. Sometimes we found ourselves laughing so hard across the miles we had to hang up, because we just couldn't talk. Normally, she could make my sides ache from laughter and cause tears of joyful stupidity to roll down my face. *But not today.*

I did not speak. I couldn't say a word.

"Irene? Is everything all right? Are you okay?" she insistently pressed for some response. I sensed her radar rising.

I could not speak, but the heartbreaking tears returned.

"Irene? You can talk to me. You know I understand . . . whatever it is. I understand. Tell me what's going on?" she urgently insisted.

Just a few minutes ago, I found my voice, but now something heavy and noxious formed in my throat. I could not dislodge it. I wanted to say something, to assure her I was all right, but no words budged past the tightness holding them back.

"Irene?" The zany one sounded serious now. "I understand. You know I understand. Say *something*."

I called her name again, forcing the suffocating weight from my throat at long last. I had no emotional energy to say anything other than her name.

"It's okay, Irene. Everything is okay," she spoke consolingly.

*Help me, Lord. Just help me.*

By sheer force of will I spoke her name once more. I *could* speak again. I needed to hoist the awful weight and throw it overboard.

"What is it? Just tell me," she pressed.

"I'm married," I moaned. The word "married" came forth in a slow, protracted upheaval. *There!* I uttered the dreadful two syllables. I could regain my voice once more, and with it, my sense of self-worth and dignity. With characteristic understanding and compassion, my jovial friend with the childlike spirit burst out laughing.

"Oh. Renie . . . girl. Oh, I'm sorry. I shouldn't be laughing. Oh, I'm so sorry. But whatever it is, laugh 'cause it ain't that serious," and she laughed uproariously again. "You know I understand. Oh, I'm sorry for laughing," and she cracked up once again.

Laughter is contagious. There is no immunity. I've been unable to resist my friend's infectious hilarity since we were girls. "You are just too stupid," I managed to say before laughing myself. "So, why are you calling me? What's so important this morning?"

"I knew God was telling me to call you. I wanted to call earlier, but I didn't want to wake you. This is just so stupid. Listen to this, and you are gonna howl."

I flipped the toilet seat lid and sat on the commode. With the phone in one hand and my chin in the other, I sat hunched over and braced myself for another crazy episode. What timing!

"You know the dinner for the pastor I told you about when you were here. Well it was last night," she began excitedly. Now, with my crisis resolved, at least temporarily, my fun-loving friend charged ahead full steam.

"You know I was planning to wear the long black skirt I showed you."

"Did you get the body suit?" I interrupted. On the subject of clothing, I could get engaged.

While in Chicago last week, Sue and I enjoyed a rare afternoon together at my friend's apartment. Talking and laughing about everything, we ate a luscious lunch our hostess prepared, then played fashion consultant as she opened her extensive closet holdings. Earlier in the day, the three of us shopped for shoes at DSW. My stylish friend found the perfect black shoes with an ornamental rhinestone buckle to complete her ensemble for the upcoming church affair. After lunch, she modeled a strapless black top she planned to wear with a floor length skirt.

"Take that off," Sue and I chorused, critiquing both the fit and appropriateness for the occasion.

Sue and my friend both own hundreds of pairs of shoes with fashionable outfits and accessories to match. I'm the fashion beggar. My paltry wardrobe is no match for that of these stylish women, but I'm learning. Sue and I both suggested a classy black body suit as the perfect complement to the elegant, formal skirt. The model struggled with the skirt's hook-and-eye closure and said she would fix it.

"Did you fix the skirt?" I asked now.

"I thought I did," she responded. "Just before the dinner ended, everyone stood to give the pastor a standing ovation. Girl, I stood up, and my skirt fell off."

"What! Are you kidding? You've got to be kidding!" I said incredulously, feeling the start of a laughter attack. I pictured this crazy woman standing in a crowded ballroom in her underwear, and I could not stop laughing. We both laughed now. My chest heaved from laughter spasms. The release felt positively marvelous.

"Girl, you are too stupid. What did you do?"

"I didn't realize what had happened at first," she explained haltingly as our laughter subsided. "I just dropped to my knees and squatted on the floor for a moment. I looked around to see who saw me," she continued. "I gathered my skirt around me as discretely as I could and just hunched over and sat back down. I was mortified," she concluded, gasping. "It was hysterical!"

We both started laughing again.

"You are insane."

"I know."

"I can't believe God had you call at just this moment," I said. "Look, I can't go into everything now. I'm getting ready for worship service. I'll call you later this afternoon when I get back." I walked out of the bathroom, crossed the room, and placed the phone in the cradle.

"What was that all about?" Amos wanted to know. That much mirth and hilarity just had to be shared. After I told him what happened, he laughed too and shook his head knowingly.

"She should have been a comedienne."

"You know, Amos, God is really merciful. How can I be upset with you and laugh at the same time? I'm going to worship service."

"I'm sorry, Irene. Please forgive me."

"Let's just talk about it later."

I returned to the bathroom and closed the door. I needed to shower. Splashing and soaping, I laughed out loud picturing this skirt wrapped around my friend's ankles in a puddle on the floor. The image of her squatting like a duck, glancing furtively around, then gathering her elegant clothing off the floor to perch surreptitiously on the nearest chair sent peels of laughter reverberating off the shower walls.

*Laughter really doeth good like a medicine, Lord. And there's no co-pay required!*

It was impossible to remain angry at my husband's insensitivity and laugh at my friend's antics at the same time. I had a choice. Later today, I'd talk with Amos. That's what the doctors always said: *Get dressed and we'll talk later,* I mused. For now, I could exercise my options.

*Father God, you are the great and mighty God. Only you could have orchestrated that phone call at just that moment. What perfect timing! Thank you for levity and laughter in the midst of a storm. You do turn sorrow into joy. Your mercies **are** new every morning. Washed clean by the blood of Jesus, all is forgiven.*

Splashing and soaping, I started to sing: *Great is thy faithfulness . . . morning by morning new mercies I see. All I have needed thy hand has provided. Great is thy faithfulness, Lord unto me!*

# Epilogue

An unknown author penned the following lines:

Cancer is so limited . . .

It cannot cripple love,
It cannot shatter hope,
It cannot corrode faith,
It cannot eat away peace,
It cannot destroy confidence,
It cannot kill friendship,
It cannot shut out memories,
It cannot silence courage,
It cannot invade the soul,
It cannot reduce eternal life,
It cannot quench the Spirit,
It cannot lessen the power
Of the resurrection.

Praise the Lord Jesus, the Author and Finisher of our faith!

Making a healthy adjustment to the long-term consequences of cervical cancer treatment has been anything but easy. Days and weeks and months without sexual intimacy are no laughing matter. Counseling sessions and therapy visits have helped to put the past in proper perspective, and the present in sharp focus. Praise God I'm alive to tell it and can yet anticipate a future of possibilities.

Life's challenges didn't stop when treatments ended. The trials and hardships are real and just kept coming. Thank God for keys to survival.

I borrowed a few pages from the family photo album to show that victorious, abundant life is possible after treatment. I will always remember our family vacation to California in August 2001. Who can forget the June 2002 celebration of God's faithfulness with nearly one hundred friends and relatives at my fifty-first birthday party? In 2003 I started speaking to women's groups about how Jesus changed my life. Now, *through Keys to Survival,* I invite an even wider audience to accept Jesus Christ as Lord and personal Savior.

To God's name be all the glory!

Charlotte, Amos, Irene, and Lorraine
in San Monica, August 2001.

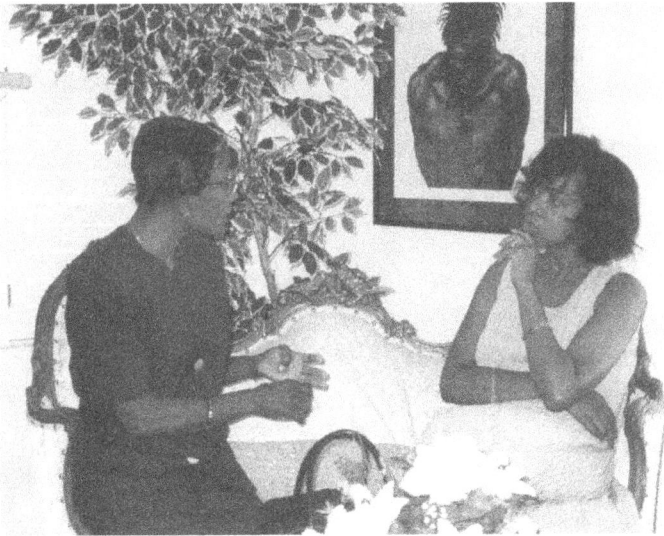

Dr. Lyra Gillette and Irene meet for the first time at
Charlotte's, August 2001.

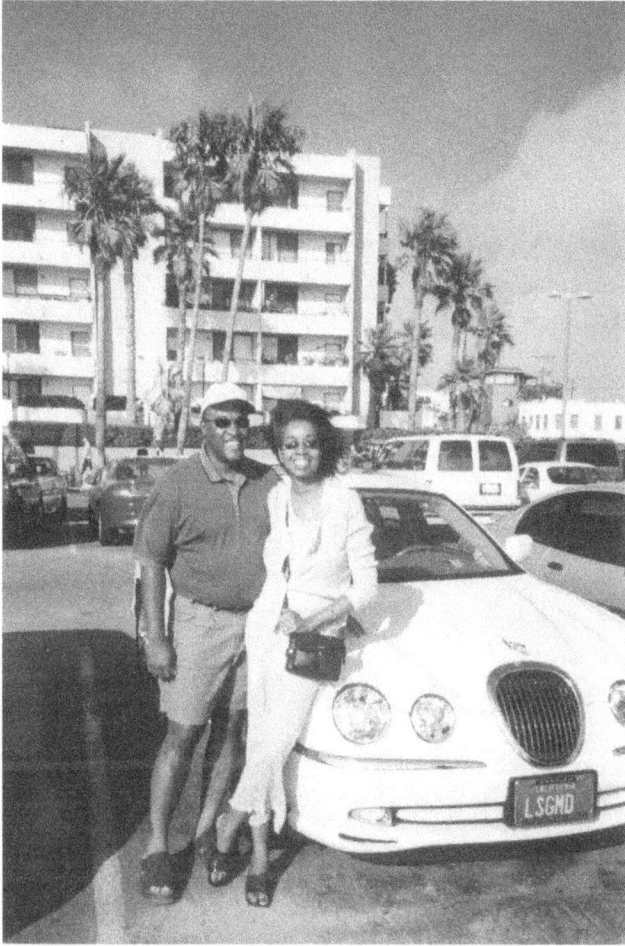

Amos and Irene at Venice Beach leaning on Lyra's Jaguar,
August 2001.  Isn't God good!

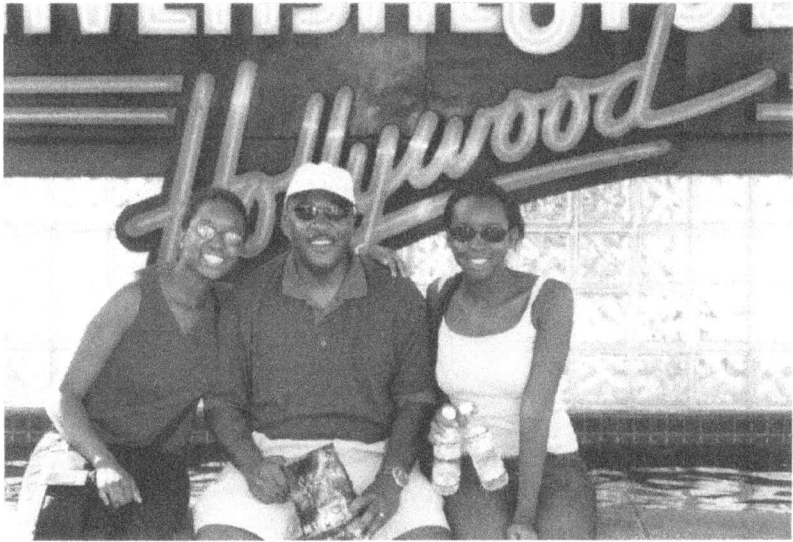

Lorraine, Amos, and Dana at Universal Studios.

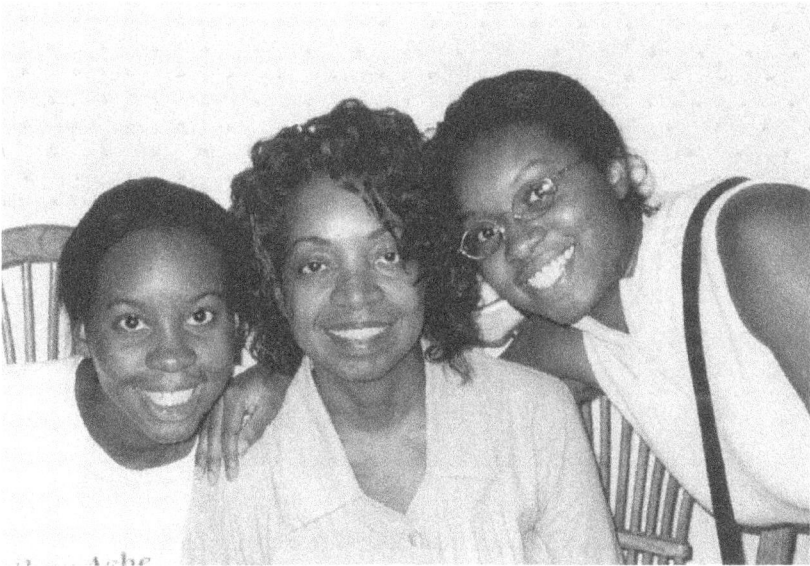

All smiles! Dana, Irene, and Lorraine, August 2001.

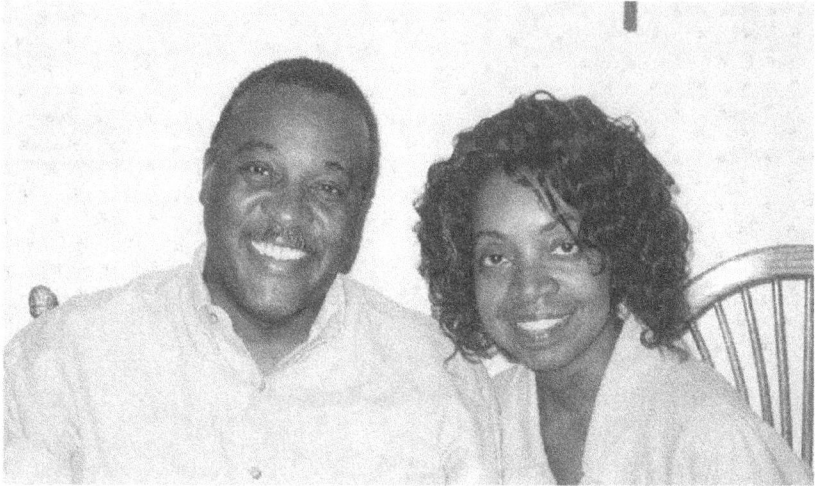

Amos and Irene relax at home after
the California vacation, August 2001.

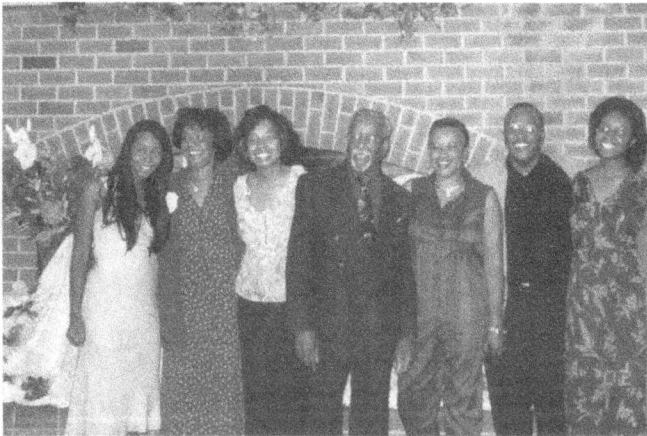

Celebrating God's faithfulness at Irene's 51st birthday
party. From left to right: Dana, Stephanie, Irene, Irene's Dad,
Susan, Amos, and Lorraine, June 2002.

# Suggested Resources*

The author highly recommends reading the Bible. If the scriptures are unfamiliar, any one of the four Gospels (the books of Matthew, Mark, Luke, and John in the New Testament) provide an excellent starting point for embracing the life and mission of Jesus Christ.

In this computer age, any topic can be researched at the touch of a key. A recent Google search uncovered nearly 6.6 million "cervical cancer" entries! By all means take an active role in understanding risk factors for disease and treatment protocols. At the same time, appreciate a website's limitations. Internet information cannot substitute for honest discussion with a trusted medical professional about one's sexual history, or regular pelvic examinations, combined with HPV and other diagnostic testing, where advised.

Every major cancer treatment center in the country offers an informational website. Selected organizations are listed below:

American Cancer Society       www.cancer.org
(800) ACS-2345

American Social Health Association   www.ashastd.org
(919) 361-8400

National Cancer Institute       www.cancer.gov
(800) 4-CANCER

National Cervical Cancer Coalition  www.nccc-online.org
(800) 685-5531

OncoLink                www.oncolink.com
(215) 349-8895

Women's Cancer Network     www.wcn.org
(800) 444-4441

Also recommended:

Henderson, Gregory S., et al. *Women at Risk: The HPV Epidemic and Your Cervical Health.* New York: Putnam Inc., 2002.


*These Internet addresses and telephone numbers were correct at the time of publication. The author assumes no responsibility for changes after publication.

## An Invitation to Write

Irene's latest book is *The Why Me Antidote: A Woman's Guide to Discovering God's Purpose, Privilege, and Potential in Adversity.* If you would like to comment on *Keys to Survival* or consider her as a speaker for your group, write to:

Irene M. Pace
c/o BTS Enterprises
P.O. Box 433
Voorhees, NJ 08043
Email: TheWhyMeAntidote@gmail.com